# UNSHAKABLE

*A Story of Resilience, Faith, Love, and Triumph*

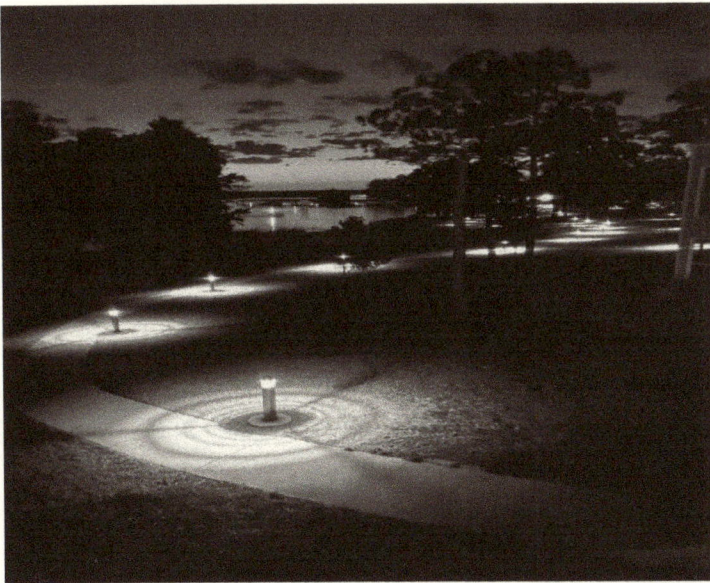

## KECHIA SCOTT

*To all the people out there on dialysis, holding onto hope for the day they receive a kidney transplant. This book is*
*a testament to your strength, fortitude, and unyielding convictions. May you find comfort in knowing you are not alone, and may your journey be filled with hope and healing.*

*With all my heart,*
*Kechia Scott*

"So do not fear, for I am with you; do not be dismayed, for I am your God. I will strengthen you and help you; I will uphold you with my righteous right hand."

—Isaiah 41:10 (NIV)
New International Version

# Contents

# Foreword

As a nephrologist who has walked alongside many patients through the labyrinth of kidney failure, I find that few journeys have been as inspiring as Kechia's. Her story is one of determination, constant belief, and the power of love and community. From the moment I met Kechia, her strength and dedication were palpable. She refused to let her diagnosis define her and instead chose to live a life filled with purpose, advocacy, and hope.

In Unshakable, Kechia doesn't just recount her experiences—she invites us into her world, sharing her trials and triumphs with raw honesty and heartfelt humor. Her ability to navigate the darkest moments with grace and to find light even in the most challenging times is a testament to the indomitable human spirit.

This book is more than a memoir; it's a guide for anyone facing adversity, a beacon for those who feel alone in their struggles, and a reminder that we can overcome even the most daunting obstacles.

Whether you are a patient, a caregiver, or someone seeking inspiration, Kechia's journey will touch your heart and empower you to face life's challenges head-on. It has been an honor to witness her journey, and I am confident that Unshakable will inspire countless others to find their strength and keep moving forward.

Dr. Muhammad Rahman
Nephrologist, DaVita Spivey

# Acknowledgments

First and foremost, I give honor and glory to God, my Lord and Savior, for His abundant blessings and for walking beside me every step of this journey. His unwavering presence has been my guiding light, my strength, and my source of sheer will and determination.

To my incredible parents—Mom and Dad—thank you for always being there, for listening, for helping whenever and wherever you could. Your love and support have been an anchor in my life, and I am forever grateful.

I extend my deepest gratitude to everyone who has walked this journey with me. To my family—your unconditional love and steadfast support have been the foundation of my strength.

To Leonardo, my rock and loyal supporter, thank you for standing by my side through every high and low, through thick and thin. Your patience, encouragement, and presence have been my source of comfort and courage, and I am endlessly thankful for you.

To my children, you are my heart, my greatest joy, and my motivation to keep moving forward—even on the toughest days. Everything I do, I do with you in mind, and I hope to always make you proud.

A heartfelt thank you to my incredible healthcare team at DaVita Spivey—Dr. Rahman, Mrs. Harris, Mrs. Earl, Ms. Mary, and Ms. Jennifer. Your dedication, care, and compassion have made an immeasurable impact on my life. You treated me not just as a patient but as a person, and I am forever grateful for your expertise and kindness.

To my incredible dialysis techs and mentors at DaVita TriCounty—Lazarus, Mrs. Shirley, Ms. Wanda, and Ms. Winsome—your guidance and belief in me have been truly unparalleled. I couldn't have navigated this journey without your wisdom, encouragement, and unwavering support. Our conversations, your instruction, and the faith you placed in me made all the difference. From the depths of my heart, you didn't just guide me—you saved my life. Thank you!

I am deeply appreciative of the National Kidney Foundation and the American Kidney Fund. Your resources, advocacy, and commitment to improving the lives of kidney patients have been a guiding light on this journey. Thank you for the vital work you do and for being a source of hope and empowerment.

To my friends, coworkers, and everyone who has offered prayers, encouragement, and support—your words and actions have lifted me in ways you may never know. Whether it was a simple check-in, a kind word, or a shared laugh, you have been part of the fabric that kept me strong and hopeful.

Lastly, to everyone living with kidney disease and those on dialysis—this book is for you. Your will to keep fighting, climbing that steep mountain, and your steadfast discipline inspire me every day. You are the true warriors, navigating life with courage and grace. I hope my story brings you the same hope and strength that your journeys have given me.

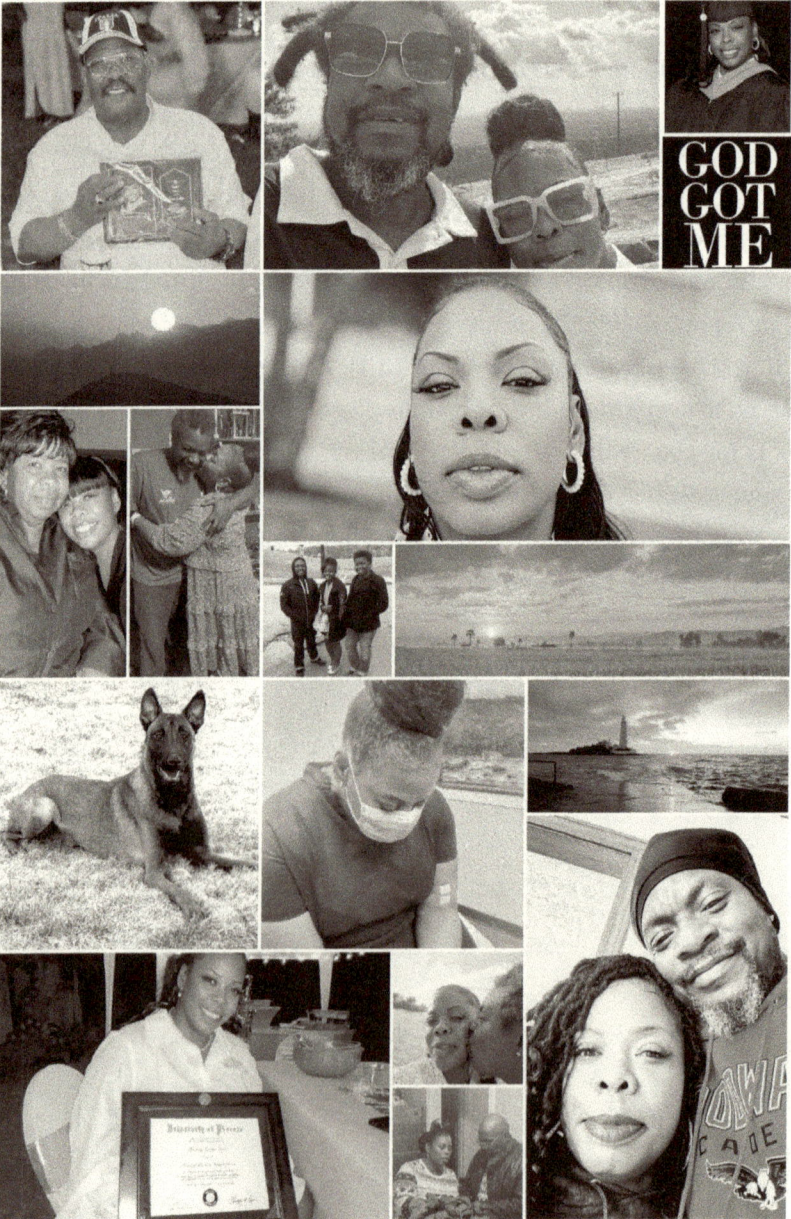

GOD
GOT
ME

# Introduction

Life has a way of testing us in ways we never expected. It presents challenges that push us to the edge, forcing us to either surrender or rise above them. Unshakable is my testimony—a story of navigating one of life's greatest trials: my battle with kidney failure and the life-changing reality of dialysis.

When I first heard the words "chronic kidney disease," I had no idea how much my world was about to change. I didn't know the exhaustion that would come from dialysis treatments, the emotional weight of waiting for a transplant, or the discipline required to maintain my health. I certainly never imagined that my journey would inspire me to write a book. Yet, here I am, sharing my story—not just as a record of survival, but as a testament to the power of faith, love, and perseverance.

This book is not just about illness—it's about resilience, strength, and the profound belief that life is still worth living, no matter the obstacles. It's about the people who stood by me— my family, my partner, my medical team, and even strangers who became unexpected sources of hope. It's about learning to laugh in the face of adversity, finding joy in the small victories, and refusing to let a diagnosis define who I am.

I wrote Unshakable for anyone who has ever faced an uphill battle and wondered if they had the strength to keep going. Whether you are fighting an illness, supporting a loved one through a difficult time, or simply searching for encouragement, I hope my story reminds you that you are not alone. You are stronger than you think, and no matter how heavy life feels, there is always a way forward.

Through every challenge, I have learned that being unshakable doesn't mean being invincible. It means standing firm when life shakes you, bending without breaking, and holding onto faith even when the future is uncertain.

There will be moments in life when you feel like giving up. When the weight of your circumstances feels unbearable, and hope seems just out of reach. But even in those moments, strength is being built within you. Every challenge you've faced has shaped you into the person you are today. And even when the road ahead feels uncertain, know that you are capable of rising above it.

If you are reading this, I want you to know—your journey matters. You matter. And no matter what you are facing, you, too, can be *Unshakable!*

# 1

# A FOUNDATION OF STRENGTH-BUILDING RESILIENCE FROM THE START

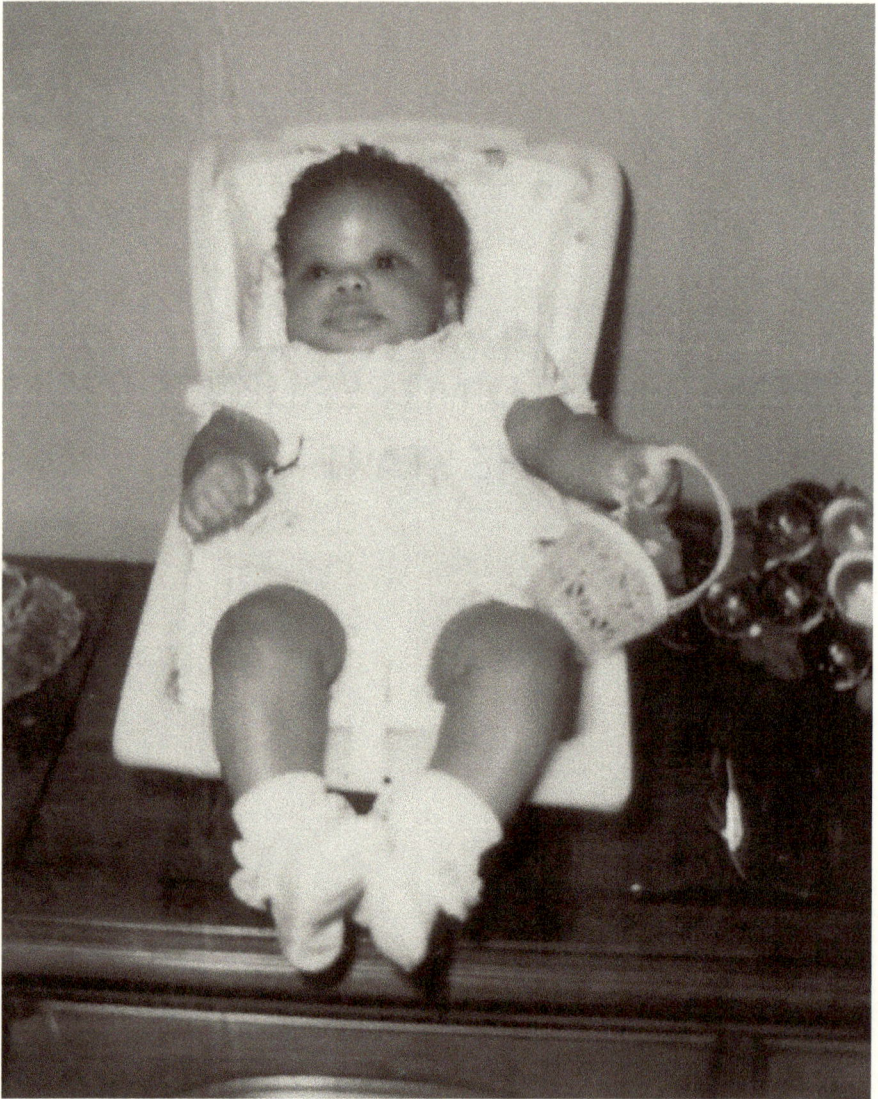

F rom the moment she entered the world, Evette Morrow was a force to be reckoned with. Born and raised in Atlanta, Georgia, she possessed a natural determination that would become the defining trait of her life. Growing up an only child, she was headstrong and inquisitive, always asking questions and seeking answers beyond what was expected of her age. She didn't just accept the world as it was—she questioned it, sought to improve it, and worked tirelessly to carve her own path.

Her journey, however, was not destined to be easy. Challenges loomed ahead— ones that would test her in ways she never imagined. Each struggle rewrote her story, not as a tale of suffering, but as proof that she was always becoming something greater.

Even in childhood, Evette displayed an exceptional work ethic. She excelled in school, never satisfied with mediocrity. Her teachers often remarked on her brilliance and dedication, predicting that she would go far in life. And she did. But her success wasn't just measured by academic and social achievement, it was fueled by an insatiable hunger for knowledge, a deep sense of purpose, and extraordinary perseverance.

Evette's spirit would soon be tested beyond her wildest expectations. Diag- nosed with end-stage renal disease, also known as kidney failure, she faced a reality that could have easily broken her spirit. Yet, instead of succumbing to despair, she pushed forward. Where others might have seen limitations, she saw opportunities. Where hardship arose, she responded with unyielding resolve.

While face a debilitating illness, Evette refused to let it dictate the trajectory of her life. She continued beyond measure—flourishing in her career, advancing her education, and never allowing her circumstances to define her. She was not just surviving; she was thriving, proving that no obstacle was greater than her will to succeed.

Evette lived in Georgia her entire life. She has worked as an educator since 2002. She has been a dedicated team member for the past seven years at Woodward Academy, the largest private school in the continental United States, located in College Park, Georgia—the very heart of where she grew up and made her mark in the world.

She loved her city—it was more than just a place; it was home. Her family and children were there, and her roller-skate community, who had embraced her since she was six years old.

Even as she navigated the demanding realities of her medical situation, Evette continued to push forward, excelling personally and professionally. She has earned her Bachelor, and Master's degrees, and is currently pursuing her Doctorate—all while undergoing dialysis treatments and managing her health with grace and dignity.

Her passion for education extends beyond the schoolhouse walls. A staunch advocate for education, she sought to create meaningful change, using her expertise to empower students in and out of her community.

This journey as an advocate for equity in education led to a monumental achievement. In December 2024, her dedication culminated in a monumental achievement—being selected as a presenter at the National Association of Independent Schools (NAIS) Annual National People of Color Conference in Denver, Colorado. Representing Woodward Academy, she hosted and led a transformative workshop titled:

***"Harnessing Data Manipulation for Equity: Empowering Students of Color in Education"***

This prestigious platform allowed Evette to share her knowledge, challenge inequities, and inspire action, demonstrating the power of data-driven advocacy in creating a more inclusive educational landscape. It was yet another testament to her grit, intelligence, and steadfast dedication to social justice, educational excellence, and personal growth—all while continuing her battle with kidney failure and dialysis.

Her story is not just one of perseverance—it is one of triumph and impact. Evette Morrow embodies the idea that life's greatest challenges do not define us; rather, how we rise above them does.

# 2

# WHEN THE BODY WHISPERS BEFORE IT SCREAMS-THE SILENT PROGRESSION OF KIDNEY DISEASE

T he body has a way of warning us when something is wrong. Sometimes, those warnings are loud and unmistakable—a stabbing pain, a fever, an injury that demands immediate attention. But other times, the warnings are whispers, so quiet and subtle that they're easy to ignore.

In hindsight, my body had been whispering for years. I just didn't know how to listen or better yet, didn't want to listen. My repetitive motto was my strength..." I feel fine!" But I wasn't. I refused to or just didn't want to believe it.

Long before I heard the words "*chronic kidney disease*", or CKD as it's affectionately known. My body had been trying to tell me something wasn't right. The signs were scattered across time like puzzle pieces I hadn't yet put together. I was always tired, but who wasn't? I had swelling in my legs and feet, but I chalked it up to long hours at work and the wrong kind of shoes. I craved ice constantly, chewing on it like my favorite snack, never realizing it was a sign of anemia.

Then there were the annual doctor's visits—the routine check-ups where they have you pee in a cup to run lab work and cultures. Year after year, my results showed protein in my urine, but I never thought much of it. It was just numbers on a chart, something my doctor noted but never emphasized. If it were serious, wouldn't they have made a bigger deal about it?

But when the protein levels continued to increase instead of decrease, and the prescription medications failed to work, my primary care physician finally referred me to a nephrologist—Dr. Muhammad Rahman, a kidney specialist in Stockbridge, Georgia.

I remember walking into his office for the first time, feeling great, completely fine. There was nothing wrong with me—at least, that's what I told myself again, and again. I wasn't sick. I wasn't in pain. I was there because my doctor told me to be.

Dr. Rahman was cordial and confident, his warm bedside manner making everything feel manageable. After reviewing my labs, he explained that I was in Stage 2 of Chronic Kidney Disease with 65% kidney function.

"*There's no need to worry,*" he assured me. "*Kidney function naturally decreases over time as we grow into adulthood.*" That was all I needed to hear. I was just like everybody else, no difference. No need to worry. I was 25 years old and felt perfectly fine—so, what was there to stress over? Before I left, Dr. Rahman gave me a few simple recommendations:

    Drink more water.
    Avoid sodas and colored drinks.
    Watch your salt intake.

It all sounded harmless, easy, like general health advice. "*Come back in six months*", he said. But six months later, I walked back into his office without making one single solitary change.

I hadn't followed his advice. Not because I was rebellious but because I still didn't think it was that serious. I was young, active, and busy—there was always something more important to focus on. But this time, when Dr. Rahman reviewed my results, his expression shifted.

*"You're now in Stage 3,"* he said. *"Your kidney function is getting worse."*

I heard the concern in his voice, but I still brushed it off. I felt fine. What did a *"stage"* even mean, anyway? As long as I wasn't sick, I had nothing to worry about. But this time was different, Dr. Rahman didn't sugarcoat it.

*"Evette, I need you to take this seriously. If you don't, you're going to end up on dialysis."*

To be honest, I didn't care. I didn't even know what dialysis was, didn't care to ask, and was the least bit concerned about learning about it. Whatever it was, it wasn't going to happen to me...so I thought.

Then, he took things a step further. He scheduled an ultrasound of my kidneys and a biopsy to rule out kidney cancer. That's when fear finally crept in. What if it was something more serious? What if I had cancer? I knew exactly what that was.

I went through the tests, waiting anxiously for the results. When they finally came back, I breathed a sigh of relief—no cancer, thank God!

But that relief was short-lived. The ultrasound revealed that one of my kidneys was significantly smaller than the other. And the good kidney? It had cysts on it.

Dr. Rahman explained what this meant—while I didn't have cancer, my kidneys weren't normal. The damage was already there, whether I felt it or not.

Still, I wasn't ready to process it. I nodded, promised to do better, and walked out of his office—without making a single change, again.

Therefore, the cycle continued. Each visit, my kidney function declined. Each warning, I ignored it. I wasn't being reckless—I just didn't believe it could happen to me. I had too much life to live, too many plans, too much to do. Kidney failure was something that happened to other people—not me.

But the body doesn't wait for you to believe. The whispers turned into murmurs. Some days, I felt an unexplained heaviness in my body, like I was moving through water instead of air. My appetite changed—sometimes I wanted everything, other times nothing at all. My skin became drier, my nails brittle. Then, at 41 years old, after evading multiple check-ups, for years, I finally walked into Dr. Rahman's office again. And this time, his expression was serious but kind, as always.

*"Evette, your kidneys are failing."*

I froze.

*"I don't understand,"* I said. *"I feel fine."*

But my lab results told a different story. My kidneys were functioning at less than 35%. I was now on the fast track to End-Stage Renal Disease (ESRD). There was no reversing it. Dialysis was no longer an *"if"* – it was a *"when."*

Denial had carried me this far, but it could take me no further. I sat motionless, staring at the medical charts, their numbers sharp and unforgiving. I wasn't sure what I was hoping to see—maybe some hidden reassurance buried in the data, some sign that I still had time. But I knew better. The truth had arrived,

11

and it refused to be softened.

I exhaled slowly, feeling the weight of it all settle on my shoulders. The long nights of exhaustion I brushed off, the tightness of my shoes, the ice cravings that I joked about but never questioned—all of it had been leading here. My body had been speaking to me, and I had turned a deaf ear. The reality was stark: my kidneys were failing. No "*maybe.*" No "*let's wait and see.*" **This was it!**

Dr. Rahman leaned forward slightly, his expression unreadable, but his eyes carried the patience of a man who had said these words before. "Your kidneys are functioning at a critical level," he said gently, but there was no mistaking the urgency in his tone. "*We need to talk about next steps.*"

Next steps? Those words sent a chill through me. Because "*next steps*" meant there was no turning back. No erasing what had already been done. No undoing the years of neglect. I wasn't just sick—I was in a fight for my life, and I had wasted too much time pretending I wasn't. This wasn't a time for tears or regrets. That wouldn't change anything now. And that's when it hit me—Dr. Rahman had been right all along. The warnings had been there for years.
In every test result.
In every swelling in my feet.
In every missed appointment.
In every moment I chose not to listen.
I had ignored it all.

Now, there were no more warnings. No more time to bargain with my body. No ignoring it. No pretending it would get better on its own. The weight of every overlooked symptom, every dismissed sign, pressed against my chest like an unbearable truth that I could no longer escape. I was faced with the stark reality staring back at me in cold, clinical terms and this time, I had no choice but to listen.

# 3

# A LIFE-CHANGING PHONE CALL–THE MOMENT EVERYTHING CHANGED

I n December 2021, during her annual winter break, Evette scheduled her routine doctor's appointments, just as she did every year. It was a habit, a precaution—something she never thought twice about. At the time, she had no symptoms, no warning signs, and felt perfectly fine. There was no fatigue beyond the usual work stress, no swelling in her feet, no discomfort. Just another year, another round of checkups, and another clean bill of health—or so she thought. Everything changed with one unexpected phone call.

She was at work, focused on the usual tasks of the day, when her phone rang. Seeing Dr. McDonald's name on the screen didn't raise any alarms. After all, routine lab results were just that—routine. But this was different. The urgency in Dr. McDonald's voice was unmistakable.

*"Evette, I need to talk to you about your lab results,"* the doctor said.

Evette barely had time to register the concern before Dr. McDonald continued, her tone firm, urgent.

*"Your creatinine levels came back at 8.12."*

Evette blinked, unsure of what to make of the number. She wasn't a doctor, and beyond knowing it was related to kidney function, the significance was lost on her. So, she responded casually, without a trace of alarm.

*"Okay."*

Dr. McDonald's voice sharpened.

*"No, you don't understand. A normal creatinine level should be between 0.5 and 1.10. Yours is dangerously high at 8.12!"*

The shift in tone sent a chill through her. It was no longer a conversation—it was a wake-up call.

Dr. McDonald's next question hit even harder.

*"Do you have a nephrologist—a kidney specialist?"*

The words confirmed what Evette had instinctively feared but never fully accepted. Her kidneys, the silent fighters in her body, had reached a breaking point. Though she had been monitored for years, the possibility of kidney failure had always felt like a distant threat. Not something that would blindside her in the middle of a workday. Not something that would upend her life in an instant.

She gave Dr. Rahman's name and contact information, still processing the weight of the moment. Before she had time to truly react, the chain of events was already unfolding.

Within an hour, just as she was gathering her things to leave work, her phone rang again.

*"Evette, this is Dr. Rahman."* His voice was steady, but there was an unmistakable urgency behind it. *"I need you to go home, pack a bag, and get to the hospital immediately. Be prepared to stay a while—because you are about to have a life-changing event."*

A life-changing event?

She sat frozen, the words echoing in her mind. Her heart pounded against her ribs, yet her body remained still. How was this happening? She felt fine. She had just wrapped up a full, productive day at work, and her evening plans were simple—some yard work with her fiance, Leonardo. Nothing about this day had suggested her world was about to be flipped upside down.

Still, she followed the doctor's instructions.

She drove home, her thoughts racing, the familiar roads blurring as she tried to process the reality crashing down on her. The moment she walked through the door and saw Leonardo, her carefully maintained composure began to crack.

She told him what the doctors had said, each word heavier than the last. His face shifted instantly—from curiosity to concern, then something deeper. A quiet fear flickered in his eyes, but he quickly masked it, inhaling slowly before exhaling in steady resolve.

There were no dramatics, no panic. Instead, Leonardo did what he did best— he stood strong beside her. He nodded, his silence a promise.

Without hesitation, they packed her belongings. The room was quiet except for the rustle of clothes and the zipping of bags. Every movement felt surreal, as if they were preparing for an unplanned trip to an unknown destination. The air between them was thick with unspoken fears, but neither allowed panic to take over. Instead, they focused on what needed to be done.

Finally, with bags in hand, they stepped into the car and drove to Piedmont Henry Hospital in Stockbridge, Georgia together.

# 4

## A COLD NIGHT IN A MUSTANG–FINDING COMFORT IN UNEXPECTED PLACES

U pon arriving at the hospital, the emergency room was a chaotic sea of patients, nurses, and exhausted staff, all overwhelmed by the relentless second wave of COVID. The air was thick with tension, muffled coughs, and the constant beeping of medical monitors. Evette clutched Leonardo's hand tighter as they approached the intake nurse, who barely looked up from her screen before delivering their options in a clipped, exhausted tone.

*"The wait is long. You can stay inside or wait in your car. We'll call your name over the PA system when it's your turn."*

Evette and Leonardo exchanged a glance. The packed waiting room was a breeding ground for illness, filled with coughing patients and the unmistakable exhaustion of overworked hospital staff. Sitting among them for hours felt like an invitation to illness, but stepping outside meant braving the bitter cold. Neither option was ideal, but at least in the car, they could isolate.

*"This way,"* Leonardo murmured, leading her back outside.

It was January 4, 2022—one of the coldest nights of the season. The wind cut through their coats like icy needles, and the parking lot, dimly lit by flickering streetlights, felt desolate. They climbed into Evette's 2014 Mustang, a car built for speed but not for comfort, and tried to settle in for what would be a long, restless night.

Hours stretched on in slow, agonizing silence.

They shifted positions constantly, trying in vain to find a comfortable way to sleep in the cramped space. The stiff leather seats provided little relief, and the freezing temperatures seeped through the windows, chilling them to the bone. They huddled in their coats, turning the engine on in short bursts just to let the heat chase away the numbness in their fingers.

At some point, exhaustion overpowered discomfort. Evette drifted in and out of a shallow sleep, her mind replaying the past 24 hours like a broken reel. Every time she opened her eyes, she saw Leonardo beside her, his breath fogging up the window as he stared out into the night, wide awake, keeping watch.

Time became meaningless. The hours blended into one another until, finally, at 9:00 AM on January 5, a voice crackled over the hospital's PA system, snapping them both back to reality.

*"Evette Morrow, please report to the front desk."*

Relief rushed through her as she and Leonardo hurried inside, rubbing their frozen hands together for warmth. But the moment they reached the check-in desk, relief turned to disbelief.

Overnight, the hospital had changed its policy—**no visitors were allowed inside.**

The words hit harder than she expected. She had braced for bad news, but not this. Not after the night they had just endured. Not after Leonardo had refused to leave her side for a single second.

Tears burned the edges of her vision as she turned to him.

"*Okay,*" she whispered, forcing her voice to stay even. "*I guess you have to take the car back home.*"

But before she could say anything else, Leonardo shook his head, his response immediate, unyielding.

"*No.*" His voice was firm, leaving no room for argument. "*We came together, and we will leave together.*"

The certainty in his words wrapped around her like a shield, pushing back the fear, the loneliness, the uncertainty.

"*I'll be in the car waiting for you until it's time to go,*" he continued, his eyes locking onto hers, full of quiet determination. "*Video call me when you get to your room.*"

Evette felt something shift inside her—a profound realization. God had been with them every step of the way and was still there. Through the uncertainty. Through the endless waiting. Through the fear that threatened to consume her. He had never left. And now, as she stood on the edge of another unknown, she could feel His presence more than ever.

Leonardo pulled her into one last embrace, holding her as if trying to transfer every ounce of strength he had left into her body. His grip was strong, yet comforting—an unspoken promise that no matter what happened next, she wouldn't face it alone.

The hospital staff gently motioned for her to come inside. She stepped back, wiping her tears quickly before turning toward the doors. As she crossed the threshold, she glanced over her shoulder one last time.

Through the glass, Leonardo was still there, watching her, standing solid, making sure she got inside safely. The morning light cast a glow behind him, outlining his silhouette—a silent guardian, waiting.

Evette pressed a trembling hand to her heart.

He was waiting for her.

And she knew, deep in her soul, that he always would.

# 5

# BEWILDERED, FINDING CLARITY THROUGH CHAOS–NAVIGATING THE UNKNOWN

O nce Evette entered the ER hospital room,she immediately video called Leonardo, just as he had requested. Their conversation bounced between serious and lighthearted topics. Leonardo asked how she was feeling, if anything had changed, and how her blood pressure was holding up? Evette, however, was more concerned about Leonardo waiting in the car. She didn't know how long she would be there and asked, *"How are you going to manage sitting in the car all day?"*

That's when they came up with a plan—they would video call throughout the day, keeping each other company, and allow their devices to charge for an hour during the least busy part of the day. Leonardo wanted to be present for every nurse's check and doctor's visit. He knew he couldn't be there if there was to be any surgery, but he wanted to stay updated on everything else.

Evette waited in the ER hospital room watching television and video calling with Leonardo for nine long hours before a hospital bed on the third floor finally became available. Leonardo was still on the video call when the nurse arrived to move her.

*"What room is she going to?"* Leonardo asked quickly.

*"Room 312 on the third floor. This is where we house our non-infectious COVID patients. Ms. Morrow will be safe there since she doesn't have COVID"* the nurse replied.

Leonardo eased the tension by telling lighthearted jokes on the way up to Room 312. When they arrived, both Evette and Leonardo thanked the nurse, keeping the video call going as she continued her duties by locking down the gurney so Evette could transition to the hospital bed.

Once she settled in Room 312, the nurse made sure Evette was comfortable. She took her vitals, checked her blood pressure, and inserted an IV line in the top of Evette's right palm.

After putting away her belongings, Evette grabbed her phone charger and Woodward Academy laptop, placing them on the hospital table where she could access them easily. Finally, she adjusted herself on the bed, turned on the TV, and propped her iPhone where Leonardo could see both her and the television screen. About an hour later, there were two firm knock at the door. Evette looked up as a handsome Indian man she had never seen before stepped inside. His jet-black hair, styled in a vintage Clark Gable swoop, framed his sharp features. Dressed in a long, flowing doctor's coat over khaki pants and what appeared to be expensive loafers, he exuded an air of confidence. Without hesitation, he raised both arms dramatically and declared...

*"Your kidneys are shot!"*

Evette, being the Capricorn that she is, immediately went on the defensive.

*"What are you talking about?"* she snapped. *"I feel fine!"* *"But you're not,"* the

doctor replied bluntly. **"You have 11% kidney function, and your creatinine level is 10.13!"**

Dang, Evette thought. It was even higher now than when Dr. McDonald had called. Her mind began to wonder if she was wrong.

Evette stared at him, confused. She had no symptoms, felt great, and couldn't understand why she was even in the hospital.

The doctor, clearly short-tempered, pointed to her laptop.

**"Since you have your computer, go to the Kidney University website and read up on kidney failure. And talk to the nurses if you don't believe me."** With that, he left the room.

Their first meeting had not gone well, but Evette wanted to understand what was happening. She took his advice and pressed the button on her remote to call the nurse. She knew God hadn't left her; He had placed the right people in her path to help her navigate this journey.

Three nurses staffed the third floor around the clock. Each shift brought in three freshly rested faces each day. The night shift nurse who responded to Evette's call was the youngest of the three—an African American woman in her late twenties or early thirties named Michelle. When she entered the room, she asked politely,

*"Yes, Ms. Morrow, how can I help you?"* *"Please, call me Evette,"* she replied, then added,

*"Can I ask you a question? And can you be totally honest with me?"*

Michelle nodded.

*"Of course."*

*"Am I really that sick? Because I sure don't feel like it."*

Michelle's eyes softened. She nodded again, this time with a nurturing expression

*"Yes, ma'am."*

Evette took a breath.

*"Can you tell me what's going on?"*

*"I'm not a doctor,"* Michelle said carefully, *"but based on what's in your chart, your kidneys have failed. You'll need dialysis to continue living."* Dr. Rahman, had never mentioned life or death before in their conversations. Needless to say, Michelle had Evette's full attention at this point.

Evette felt a weight settle in her chest.

*"What's dialysis? Can you explain it to me?"* asked Evette.

Michelle explained gently, *"It's a treatment that removes waste and excess fluid from your blood when your kidneys can't do it anymore. Without it, life expectancy is not likely or very short."*

Hearing it from Michelle, with her soft, reassuring voice, made the reality sink in. Evette asked about the Kidney University website and Michelle stayed with her, navigating the site and answering questions. By the time Michelle left, Evette understood—her doctor, the nephrologist, was right, even if his bedside manner needed serious work.

The following Wednesday, the doctor returned. This time, he was less dramatic, and Evette had done her homework. She greeted him with an apology, thanking him for giving her the time to process everything.

Dr. Toonde smiled and admitted, "*I could've handled our first meeting better.*"

As they continued, Leonardo stayed on the video call as the doctor outlined the next steps—starting with the port catheter surgery. He explained that the port would be used to remove the "*bad*" blood and return the "*clean*" blood to her body. The port would remain until a graft or fistula, which was the gold standard for dialysis, was placed in her arm. He emphasized that the port catheter was temporary and could not get wet because it was prone to infection. Once the port catheter was inserted, the doctor explained, they would begin a round of dialysis for four hours each day at the hospital to ensure it was functioning properly. They also wanted to monitor closely to see if Evette's kidneys would regenerate.

"*Which hand is dominant?*" the doctor asked.

"*The right,*" Evette replied.

"*Then we'll place the fistula in your left arm.*"

While researching online, Evette mentally prepared herself for the port catheter procedure but grew increasingly apprehensive about the fistula after seeing images on the internet. The photos were unsettling—showing bulging, disfigured veins that looked both painful and unattractive. Unlike the port catheter, which could be easily hidden beneath her clothes, the fistula was typically placed on the inside of the upper arm, making it difficult to conceal. Evette dreaded the thought of having to wear long-sleeve blouses for the rest of her life just to cover the unsightly lump on her inner forearm.

Before leaving, Dr. Toonde informed Evette that she couldn't be discharged until she had a spot at a dialysis center. He recommended the DaVita TriCounty

Dialysis Center, where he oversaw patient care.

*"Our staff is exceptional, and we average at least one kidney transplant per month,"* he added.

Evette agreed, thanking him for his help. Once he left, she felt a sense of relief. They had finally connected, and she now understood her condition. She discussed everything with Leonardo before settling in to do some work for Woodward Academy.

Bewildered no more.

# 6

# THE DIAGNOSIS HAS A NAME–UNDERSTANDING THE ENEMY

After further review of her kidneys, Dr. Toonde diagnosed Evette with Focal Segmental Glomerulosclerosis (FSGS), a kidney disease marked by the scarring (sclerosis) of certain parts (segments) of the glomeruli. These tiny filters in the kidneys remove waste and excess fluid from the blood, keeping the body balanced and functioning properly. When damaged, they lose efficiency, leading to protein leakage into the urine, a condition known as nephrotic syndrome. Over time, the disease progresses, chipping away at kidney function until dialysis or a transplant becomes inevitable.

The diagnosis came with a mix of emotions. On one hand, finally knowing what she was dealing with was a relief. No more ambiguity, no more dismissive reassurances from doctors who had previously told her she was "*probably just dehydrated.*" But with that relief came fear—the gut-wrenching kind that gnawed at the edges of her mind, whispering all the what-ifs she wasn't ready to face. What if this was her life now? What if things got worse? What if there was no miracle waiting for her?

Dr. Toonde walked her through the reality of FSGS: swelling in the legs and feet, chronic fatigue, high blood pressure, and an ever-present battle to keep her body functioning as normally as possible. As he spoke, Evette sat in silence, absorbing his words—but deep down, she already knew.

Because she had been living with these symptoms for months.

The exhaustion that made getting out of bed feel like a marathon. The swelling in her legs and ankles that she chalked up to "too much salt" or "bad circulation." The sky-high blood pressure readings she ignored because, in her mind, she was "too young" for anything serious. The brain fog that made simple tasks feel overwhelming. All of it had been screaming for her attention, warning her that something was deeply wrong. But she had been too stubborn, too dismissive, too unwilling to believe that her body could betray her like this.

For so long, she had convinced herself that it wasn't that bad if she drank more water, and cut back on certain foods. She told herself that she just needed more sleep, less stress, maybe a vacation—anything but the truth. Because accepting that something was wrong meant accepting that she wasn't in control. And Evette had spent her whole life fighting for control.

But there was no running from it now.

For the first time, she was truly present, hanging onto every word Dr. Toonde said. She asked the questions she had once been too afraid to say out loud:

"How fast does it progress?"

"Will I need a transplant?"

"How long do I have to be on dialysis?"

Dr. Toonde didn't sugarcoat the truth. FSGS was unpredictable—some patients stabilized with treatment, while others declined rapidly. A transplant was a possibility, but not a guarantee. Dialysis is necessary, and how soon depends on how well her body responds to medication, treatment, and lifestyle changes. It was a hard conversation, but one she needed to hear.

Back in her hospital room, the weight of reality pressed down on her. The memories of those appointments with Dr. Rahman flooded back—the warnings, the concerned looks, the repeated instructions she had brushed off as overcautious. She had been stubborn, convinced she had more time, that her body would somehow fix itself. But it hadn't. And now, the consequences of her choices had caught up to her. If only she had listened. If only she had taken his words seriously. She had gambled with her health, and now, she was paying the price—with her freedom, her independence, and the life she once knew.

Evette had always been strong. Self-pity wasn't in her nature, and even if it had been, something around her wouldn't allow her to sink into it. She knew what it was—God's presence, firm and ever-present, refusing to let her spiral. So, she gathered herself. She took a deep breath, wiped away the lingering tears, and opened her laptop.

If she couldn't change the past, she could at least arm herself with knowledge.

She dove into research, combing through medical studies, patient testimonials, and scientific articles about FSGS. The more she read, the more unsettling the reality became. There was no cure. The available treatments focused on slowing the disease, not reversing it. Some patients managed to control their symptoms for years, even decades. Others weren't as fortunate.

Still, she needed more than just clinical explanations—she needed to hear from people who had lived it. She found online communities filled with stories that mirrored her own: people who had ignored their symptoms, convinced themselves they were fine, only to wake up one day and realize they weren't.

Some had found ways to navigate life despite the setbacks, adapting to the limitations with grit and optimism. Others were barely holding on, trapped in an endless cycle of doctor visits, insurance battles, and transplant waitlists that stretched on for years.

Evette couldn't hide from the truth any longer. She had spent too much time pretending she was invincible, convincing herself that whatever was happening to her body wasn't serious. That she was different. That she had time. But now, sitting in a hospital bed with her kidneys failing, she felt the full weight of her choices.

Leonardo saw it too.

*"We'll get through this,"* he reassured her during a late-night video call, his face illuminated by the soft glow of his phone screen. *"One step at a time."*

His voice was calm, steady—but she could see the worry in his eyes. He had been warning her for months, noticing the changes she refused to acknowledge. The swelling. The exhaustion. The blood pressure readings that should have been a wake-up call. He had begged her to take it seriously, to listen to her body. She hadn't. And now, here they were.

As the days passed, something inside her shifted. The fear was still there, lingering beneath the surface, but something stronger was beginning to take its place. Not just the will to survive—but the determination to take charge. Real control. Of her health. Of her choices. Of her future. She couldn't undo the past. She couldn't rewrite the moments when she had ignored the warnings.

But she could decide what happened next.

Still, there was no escaping the reality of her situation.

Her father had experienced kidney failure in 2008, but his story had been different. His kidneys had healed. After just ten rounds of dialysis, his body had recovered, allowing him to leave the hospital with a second chance. His struggle had been temporary.

Hers wasn't.

There would be no miraculous recovery. No sudden turnaround. Her kidneys would not regenerate. Dialysis wasn't a short-term inconvenience—it was a lifeline, one she would depend on for the foreseeable future. A bridge to a transplant that might take years to happen—if it happened at all.

And yet, knowing all of this, she refused to crumble.

She wouldn't let this disease define her, but she wouldn't ignore it anymore either. She had made peace with the truth—this was her new reality. But it didn't have to be the thing that broke her.

Her story wasn't about what she had lost.

It was about what she was ready to fight for.

# 7

# A VIRTUAL JOURNEY TOGETHER–LOVE ACROSS THE DISTANCE

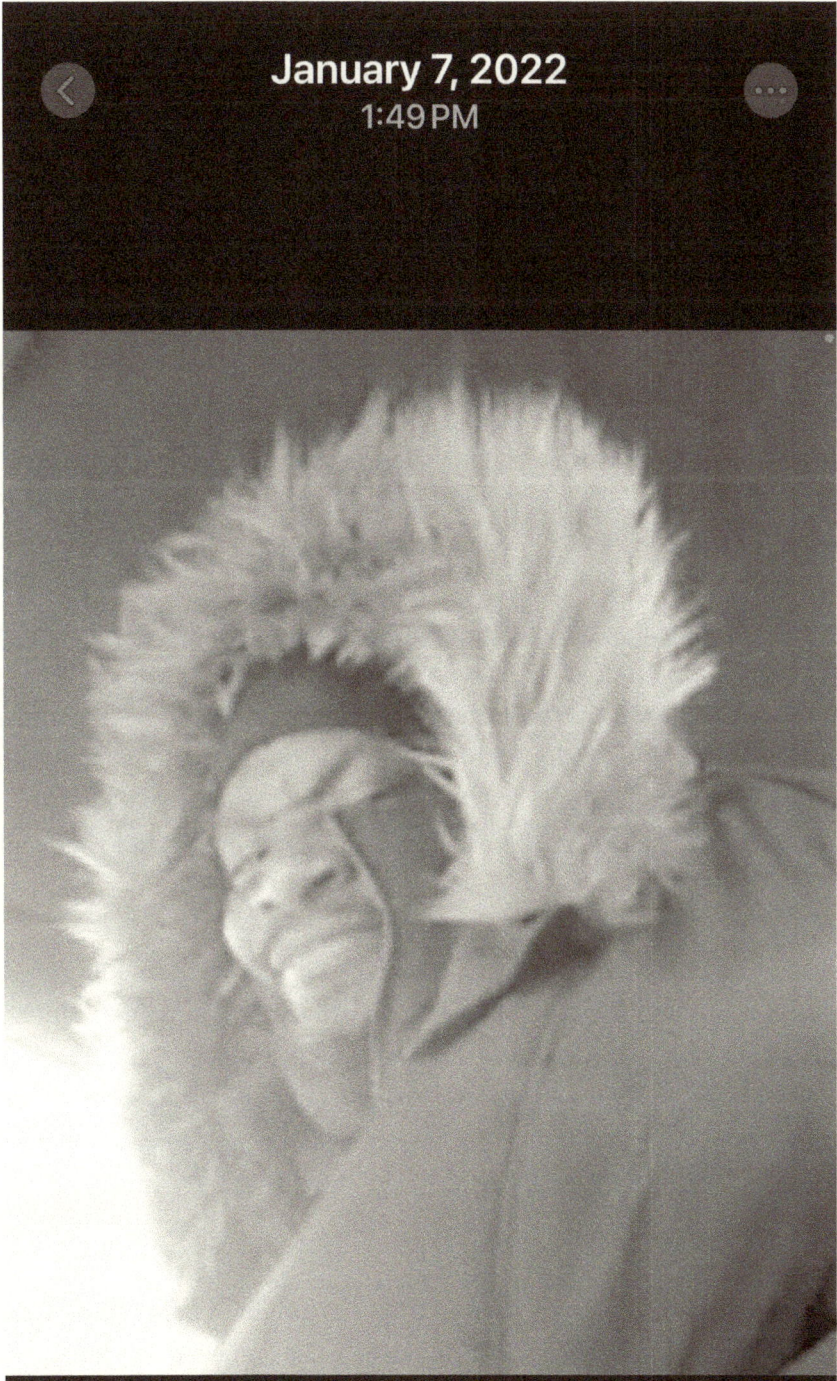

January 7, 2022
1:49 PM

For the next eight days, Evette remained in the hospital, her world reduced to the sterile walls of her room, the rhythmic beeping of machines, and the quiet shuffling of nurses checking vitals. Yet, despite the IV lines, the endless blood draws, and the exhaustion that clung to her like a heavy fog, she refused to surrender to idleness.

From her hospital bed, she continued working remotely on her school-issued laptop, juggling her responsibilities at Woodward Academy while keeping up with her coursework at the University of Phoenix. Emails were answered, deadlines were met, and assignments were submitted, all while her body battled against her own failing kidneys. She refused to let her condition dictate her productivity, determined to hold on to whatever fragments of normal life she could salvage.

Though she had informed the President, Vice President, and her supervisor about her hospitalization, she couldn't bring herself to share the news with her colleagues. A mix of pride and quiet shame kept her from broadcasting her reality. She didn't want pity, didn't want hushed whispers about her health to define her presence at the Academy. Instead, she asked that her situation remain confidential. They respected her wishes, agreeing to keep the details private.

But even as she maintained her work ethic, she knew she couldn't power through school on sheer will alone. Acknowledging the road ahead, she reached out to the Office of Student Affairs at the University of Phoenix to request academic accommodations. The response was swift—within days, her request was approved, granting her the flexibility needed to continue her coursework without jeopardizing her health. It was a relief, a small victory in the midst of uncertainty.

Despite the upheaval, Evette refused to let the weight of her circumstances dull her spirit. Even confined to a hospital bed, she remained the same quick-witted, lighthearted presence she had always been. She cracked jokes with the nurses, found humor in the absurdity of her situation, and made it her mission to keep those around her smiling. Laughter echoed down the hospital halls, an unexpected contrast to the sterile, somber environment. It wasn't just for the sake of others—it was for herself. Humor had always been her shield, and now, it became her lifeline.

But while Evette found ways to maintain her sense of self, Leonardo refused to leave her side—at least, as close as the hospital rules allowed him to be.

True to his word, he never left the parking lot. Night after night, he remained stationed in the Mustang, unwilling to stray too far. He braved the freezing temperatures with nothing but the heat from the car's vents and the layers of blankets he had stashed in the backseat. When the battery eventually gave out, the paramedics who had come to know him well jumped his car, allowing him to keep warm during the brutal winter nights.

His devotion did not go unnoticed. The hospital staff whispered about him, touched by the rare sight of unwavering commitment. Nurses who checked on Evette at night often saw the soft glow of her video call screen illuminating his sleeping face, his steady breathing a quiet comfort on the other end of the line. They would smile, nudging her playfully.

"*He really loves you,*" one of them remarked, shaking her head in admiration. "*We rarely see this kind of devotion.*"

Leonardo's presence became something of a legend within those walls—a tale of love and loyalty that softened even the most hardened hearts.

Then came January 10, 2022.

The day everything changed.

After days of uncertainty, Evette was wheeled into surgery to have a dialysis port catheter placed near the right side of her collarbone. The ride down the cold, dimly lit hospital corridor felt surreal. As the ceiling lights flickered past her, she tried to process the weight of what was happening. There was no turning back now.

The operating room was stark, the overhead surgical lights casting an almost blinding glare. The last thing she remembered before slipping under anesthesia was the sound of muffled voices, the sterile scent of antiseptic, and the quiet hum of machines preparing to take over.

When she awoke, the fog of anesthesia clung to her like a heavy curtain, dulling the pain but not the reality of what had just been done to her body. She reached for her collarbone instinctively, fingers brushing against the foreign presence of the catheter. It was real. A blue and red plastic line now protruded from her chest, embedded beneath the skin—a permanent reminder that her life had changed.

This wasn't temporary.

There was no quick fix, no short-term inconvenience she could power through. Dialysis was now a part of her, woven into her existence. The weight of it all threatened to suffocate her, pressing down on her chest, making it hard to breathe.

Then, through the haze of discomfort, Leonardo's voice broke through.

"*Count your blessings,*" he murmured softly through the phone. "*It could have been worse. You're here. You're alive.*"

She swallowed the lump in her throat. He was right. It could have been worse.

She took a slow, measured breath and closed her eyes.

Yes, her life had changed. Yes, the road ahead would be long, filled with challenges she had yet to fully comprehend. But she wasn't facing it alone. She had Leonardo. She had her faith. She had the same fire within her that had carried her through every battle before this one.

God was still with her.

And with that realization, she made a choice.

She wasn't going to sink. She wasn't going to let this define her.

This was just another chapter in her story.

And she would face it—head-on, determined, and fearless.

# 8

# A NEW NORMAL–ADAPTING TO LIFE WITH DIALYSIS

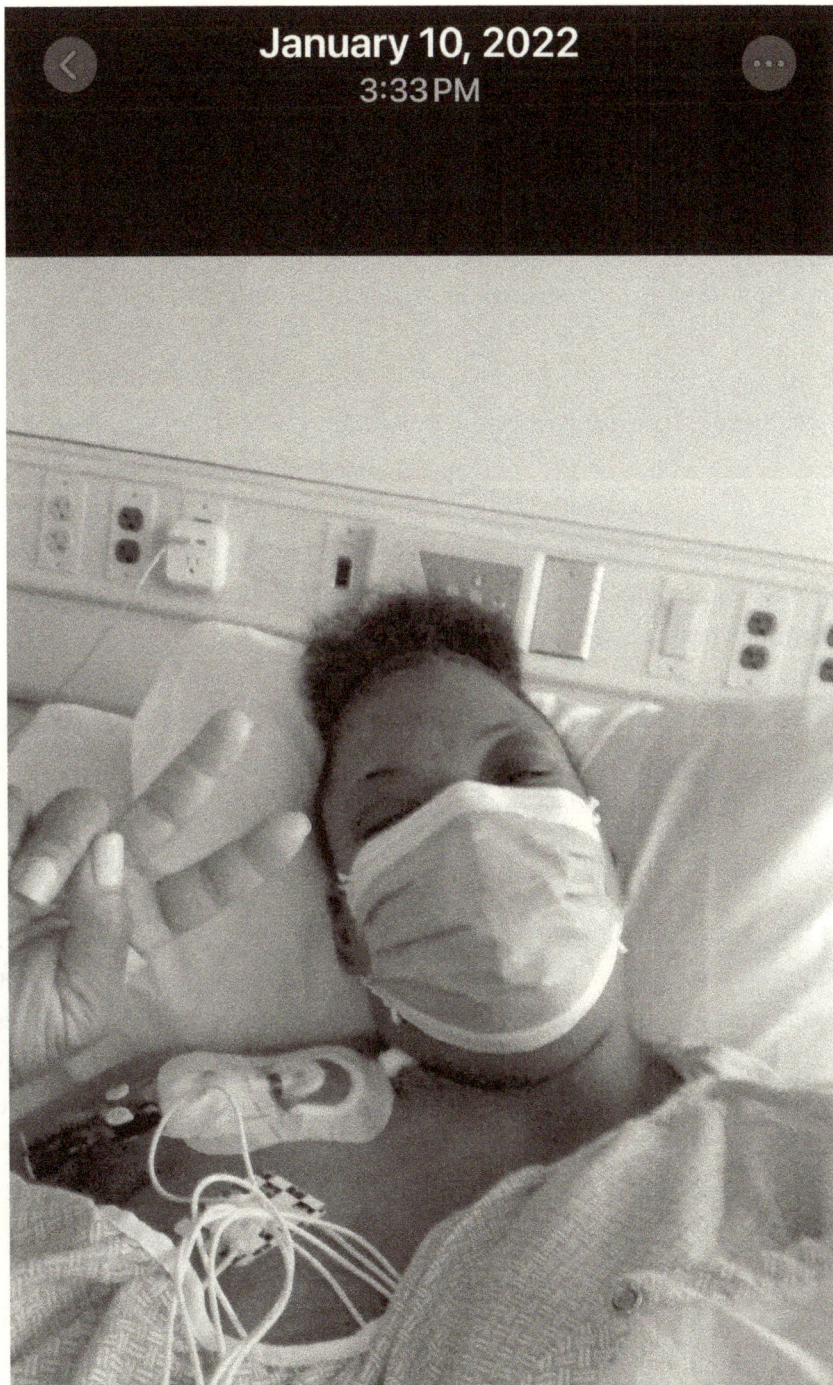

January 10, 2022
3:33 PM

After being discharged from the hospital, Evette stepped into a world that felt both familiar and entirely foreign. The walls of her home were the same, but everything else had changed. Dialysis was no longer a stopgap—it was now a new addition to her body and her life. Her days, once filled with spontaneous plans, aspirations, and the easy rhythm of daily routines, were now structured around treatment schedules, strict dietary restrictions, and a growing calendar of medical appointments.

Her life had been turned upside down. Only showing remnants of the past and how she wished she had listened to Dr. Rahman's instructions.

The first few weeks at home felt surreal. Every corner of her house seemed to reminders of the life she used to live—one without machines dictating her mornings or medications lining her kitchen counters. Yet, Evette was determined to find balance in this new reality.

While her circumstances had shifted dramatically, her spirit remained unshaken. She approached her new normal with the same grit that had carried her through the darkest days in the hospital, refusing to let her illness define her.

One unexpected transformation was physical. The weight she had lost during her hospital stay left her looking more radiant than she could have anticipated. Friends and family commented on her glowing skin and renewed energy, even if that energy came in waves. This physical shift became a small but powerful reminder that even in the midst of hardship, there could be unexpected light. It was as if her body, though weakened in some ways, was also revealing a new kind of strength—one that reflected both her inner fortitude and her ability to adapt.

Her mornings began earlier than ever before. By 4:30 AM, Evette was awake, preparing for her 5:00 AM dialysis sessions. These treatments were grueling, testing both her physical limits and her mental resolve. Yet, a midst the exhaustion and discomfort, there was comfort in the routine. Knowing exactly what to expect—what the machines would do, how her body might react— offered a strange sense of control. And then there was Leonardo. His presence outside the dialysis center, waiting patiently in his car during every session, became her silent source of strength. Just knowing he was there, no matter the weather or the hour, made the entire experience feel less isolating. Balancing work with her treatment schedule was no small feat. Yet, Evette managed to maintain her full-time role at Woodward Academy, much to the admiration of her colleagues. They marveled at her vigor, often expressing disbelief at how she could juggle the demands of her job while enduring such intense medical treatments. But for Evette, work wasn't just about fulfilling responsibilities or earning a paycheck—it was a symbol of normalcy. It was proof that she was still capable, still strong, and still herself regardless of everything she was facing.

Dietary changes quickly became another crucial part of her new reality. Foods she once enjoyed were now off-limits. She had to monitor her fluid intake meticulously, avoid high-phosphorus foods, and stick to strict sodium limits. This constant vigilance felt like a battle, but Evette approached it with her characteristic humor. She often joked about her "newfound relationship" with bland meals and unsalted snacks, finding laughter even in the restrictions.

Her social life also required adjustments. Spontaneous outings, roller skating, fishing trips, and late-night gatherings— her favorite hobbies—now had to be carefully planned. Every detail mattered: Did she have enough energy to participate? Could she manage her fluid restrictions while out? Amid these hurdles, Evette refused to let dialysis limit her joy. She found creative ways to stay connected with friends and family, often hosting small gatherings at home where she felt most comfortable and in control.

Emotionally, the journey was a roller coaster. There were days filled with frustration, moments when the weight of her reality felt overwhelming. The constant monitoring, the strict schedules, the ever-present fatigue—it all felt like too much at times. But through it all, Evette's spirituality remained her anchor. She leaned on prayer, drawing strength from her spiritual practices and her belief that God had a purpose for her journey. Even in her darkest moments, she found light in the belief that she was not walking this path alone.

And, of course, Leonardo's support never wavered. His presence wasn't just physical; it was emotional and spiritual. He became her confidant, her advisor, her rock. Their bond deepened in ways neither of them could have anticipated, proving that love could flourish even in the most challenging of circumstances.

As the months passed, what once felt foreign began to feel familiar. The routines, the restrictions, the treatments—they all became part of the fabric of her life. The fear that had loomed large in the beginning started to fade, replaced by a quiet confidence. Evette embraced her new normal, not as a limitation but as an opportunity to showcase her durability and vigor. She was living proof that life could still be beautiful and fulfilling, even with its unexpected twists and turns.

Her story wasn't just about surviving kidney failure—it was about succeeding despite it. Evette's journey became a testament to the power of triumphing over adversity. And as she continued to navigate this new chapter, she did so with grace, humor, and an unbreakable spirit.

# 9

# DIALYSIS & TRIUMPH: RECLAIMING LIFE–TURNING STRUGGLES INTO STRENGTH

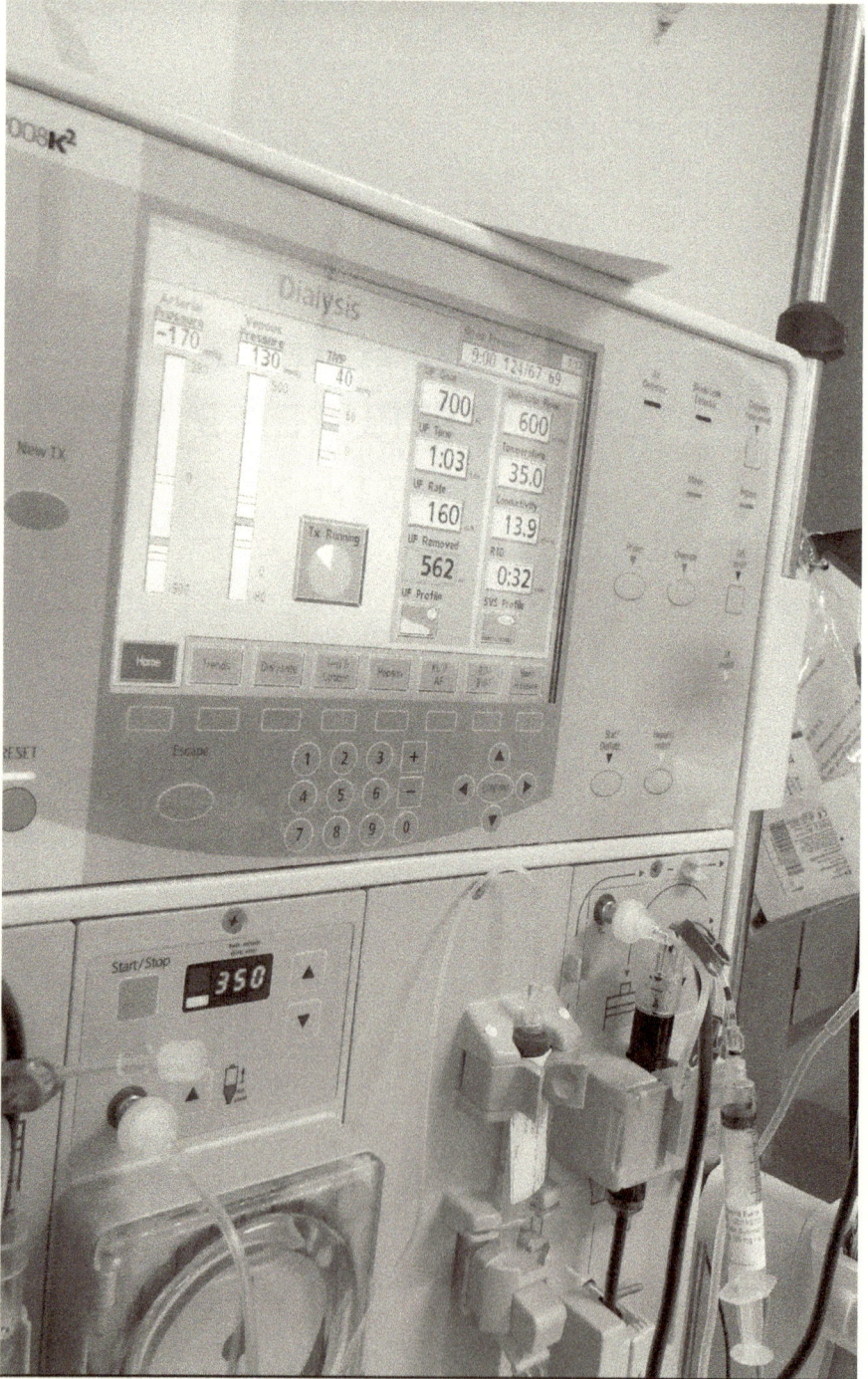

With her hospital stay behind her, Evette faced the next phase of her journey head-on—dialysis at DaVita TriCounty Dialysis Center. Every Tuesday, Thursday, and Saturday at 5:00 AM, she arrived for her sessions, tethered to a machine for three hours and forty-five minutes. This routine wasn't temporary; it was her new reality. But instead of allowing it to dictate her life, Evette was determined to master it.

After spending one week working remotely from her hospital bed and three weeks working remotely from home, Evette transitioned back into her routine. On the days when she wasn't feeling up to remote work, she utilized Intermittent Family Medical Leave (FMLA) to give herself the necessary space to recover. Once she found her footing, Evette returned to Woodward Academy, determined to reclaim her sense of normalcy and purpose.

She dove back into her responsibilities with the same vigor that had defined her before her diagnosis. To her colleagues, it seemed almost impossible— how could someone undergoing such grueling treatments continue to perform at such a high level? But for Evette, work was more than just a job. It was her way of proving to herself and the world that she was still capable, still strong.

Beneath her determined exterior, however, dialysis was no gentle process. Unlike the machines in the hospital, which had been softer and more forgiving, the in-center dialysis machines were aggressive and unrelenting. Evette quickly realized that her body needed time to adjust to the harshness of these treatments. Each session pushed her to her limits.

There were days when the machines would remove too much fluid, causing her blood pressure to plummet dangerously low. When that happened, it felt as though her spirit was floating above her body, leaving her immobilized for hours. Recovering from these episodes wasn't as simple as resting or taking a nap. It required complete stillness, allowing her body to recalibrate and regain its strength naturally.

Then came the cramps—sharp, debilitating, and unlike anything she had ever experienced. These weren't ordinary muscle cramps. They seized her body with such intensity that she felt paralyzed, unable to move or even cry out. Imagine the worst Charley horse imaginable, multiplied by ten—that's what dialysis cramps felt like. They struck without warning, leaving her gasping in pain until they finally, mercifully, subsided.

At every treatment, a saline bag hung nearby as a safety net for moments when her blood pressure dropped too low. A quick release of saline would bring immediate relief, restoring her equilibrium. But for the cramps, there was no quick fix. She had to endure them, lying there motionless, waiting for the pain to pass. It was a brutal reminder that while she could control many aspects of her treatment, some battles had to be fought with sheer willpower.

But Evette was nothing if not a quick learner. She realized that surviving dialysis wasn't just about enduring the treatments—it was about mastering them. She learned to manage her fluid intake meticulously, avoiding the pitfalls that could lead to dangerous drops in blood pressure. She followed her dietary guidelines with discipline, understanding that every choice she made outside the dialysis chair impacted how her body responded inside it. She listened to her body, adjusting her routines to find the delicate balance between treatment and recovery.

Her drive didn't go unnoticed. At Woodward Academy, her dedication and strength were recognized and celebrated. The administration made accommodations to support her journey, allowing her to work full-time with half-days on Tuesdays and Thursdays to accommodate her dialysis schedule. This flexibility was more than just a professional courtesy—it was a lifeline, a way for Evette to maintain her sense of purpose and normalcy. It allowed her to continue advancing in her career while managing the demands of her health.

Through it all, Evette found herself not just surviving but reclaiming her life.

Dialysis was no longer an insurmountable obstacle; it was a challenge she had learned to navigate with God and grace. She discovered that even in the face of physical limitations, she could find strength and fulfillment. She was not defined by her illness but by her ability to rise above it.

Her journey became a testament to the power of perseverance. Each session, each challenge, each victory was a reminder that she was stronger than she had ever imagined. Dialysis had entered her life as an unwelcome guest, but Evette had turned it into an opportunity—a chance to demonstrate her persistence, to prove that even in the face of life's toughest battles, she was *unshakable*.

# 10

# THE DIALYSIS COMMUNITY–FINDING FAMILY IN UNLIKELY PLACES

W alking into the dialysis center each morning, Evette began to notice something—she was not alone. The room was filled with people of all ages and backgrounds, each navigating their own battles with kidney failure. Some patients were talkative, sharing stories of their lives before illness, while others sat quietly, eyes closed, as the machines hummed around them, filtering their blood and sustaining their lives. The rhythmic beeping of the machines became a strange symphony, underscoring both the fragility and stamina of life.

As the days passed, Evette observed something else— many of the patients didn't look like her. Some were amputees due to diabetes, others were paraplegic, and many couldn't walk unassisted. While Evette and Leonardo drove to the center each day, many patients relied on medical transportation. Ambulances frequently arrived to transfer those whose blood pressure was too high or who had retained excessive fluid, leading to vision problems, heart palpitations, or shortness of breath. These daily emergencies were a stark reminder of how precarious life on dialysis could be.

An unspoken rule governed at the center: if a patient missed a session, they couldn't return without first visiting the hospital and presenting discharge papers first. No technician wanted to risk being responsible for a patient's decline, so they strictly adhered to protocols. This reinforced the gravity of every session, emphasizing the necessity of consistency and vigilance.

Amid the sterile walls and mechanical sounds, Evette found warmth in the people surrounding her. She drew comfort from the silent understanding shared among those who faced the same daily battle. The dialysis center wasn't just a place for treatment—it became a network of empathy and mutual support. One of the most influential figures in this space was Lazarus, a seasoned dialysis technician known for his calming presence. He had an innate ability to put patients at ease, offering words of encouragement and practical advice with each session.

His steady demeanor made the intimidating environment feel a little less overwhelming.

*"Don't worry,"* he told Evette on her first morning in the chair. *"I'll teach you everything you need to know about this journey. You're going to be just fine."*

Lazarus did exactly what he said, he became more than just a technician— he became her mentor. He guided Evette through the intricacies of dialysis: managing fluid intake, maintaining stable numbers, and understanding the subtle messages her body sent. His guidance wasn't just technical but an emotional anchor, giving Evette a sense of control over her health.

*"All I ask is for you to trust me and follow my recommendations,"* he'd say with a confident smile. And trust him, she did.

Evette's support system extended beyond Lazarus. Mrs. Shirley, Ms. Winsome, and Ms. Wanda, three additional dedicated technicians, brought nurturing spirits to the center. They often encouraged Evette to explore home dialysis, describing the freedom and flexibility it could offer. It was Ms. Wanda who first suggested meeting with the home dialysis nurse during a future visit to TriCounty—a suggestion that planted a seed for a pivotal decision in Evette's journey.

Mrs. Shirley was a steady source of support, always encouraging Evette to consider home dialysis, convinced it would be a perfect fit for her. She frequently took the time to sit with Evette, engaging in conversations that ranged from dialysis to life in general. Evette felt a deep connection with Mrs. Shirley, as she reminded her of her close friends—someone who would naturally belong in their circle.

Then, there was Ms. Winsome, whose no-nonsense attitude balanced the compassion of Lazarus, Mrs. Shirley, and Ms. Wanda. She was firm yet fair, pushing Evette to take full ownership of her health. Ms. Winsome was the first to teach Evette about self-cannulation and always had a gentle touch with the needle. Her straightforward approach provided a different kind of support, empowering Evette to face the realities of her condition head-on.

But it wasn't just the staff who shaped Evette's experience. She began to form bonds with fellow patients—people who understood her struggles in ways even her closest friends and family couldn't. They exchanged stories of life before kidney failure, shared their fears about the future, and celebrated the small victories that kept them moving forward. Their connection was unspoken but undeniable—a silent acknowledgment that while their paths were unique, their fight was shared.

Over time, the dialysis center became more than just a place of treatment; it became a second family. Patients celebrated each other's milestones, offered comfort during setbacks, and even found joy in the mundane routines tethered to their machines. Thanksgiving meals were shared, games played on special occasions, and laughter echoed in unexpected moments. In this space, Evette discovered not just purpose but also a sense of belonging. They weren't just surviving—they were living, finding moments of connection and hope amidst the challenges.

Through Lazarus's mentorship, Ms. Wanda and Mrs. Shirley's encouragement, Ms. Winsome's firm guidance, and the camaraderie of her fellow
patients, Evette learned to navigate dialysis with confidence. What once felt
like a place of fear and uncertainty transformed into a space of empowerment
and growth. Here, in the most unlikely of places, she discovered the profound
strength that comes from shared experiences—a reminder that even in life's
most daunting challenges, she was never truly alone.

# 11

# TAKING CONTROL: THE HOME DIALYSIS JOURNEY–EMPOWERING THROUGH INDEPENDENCE

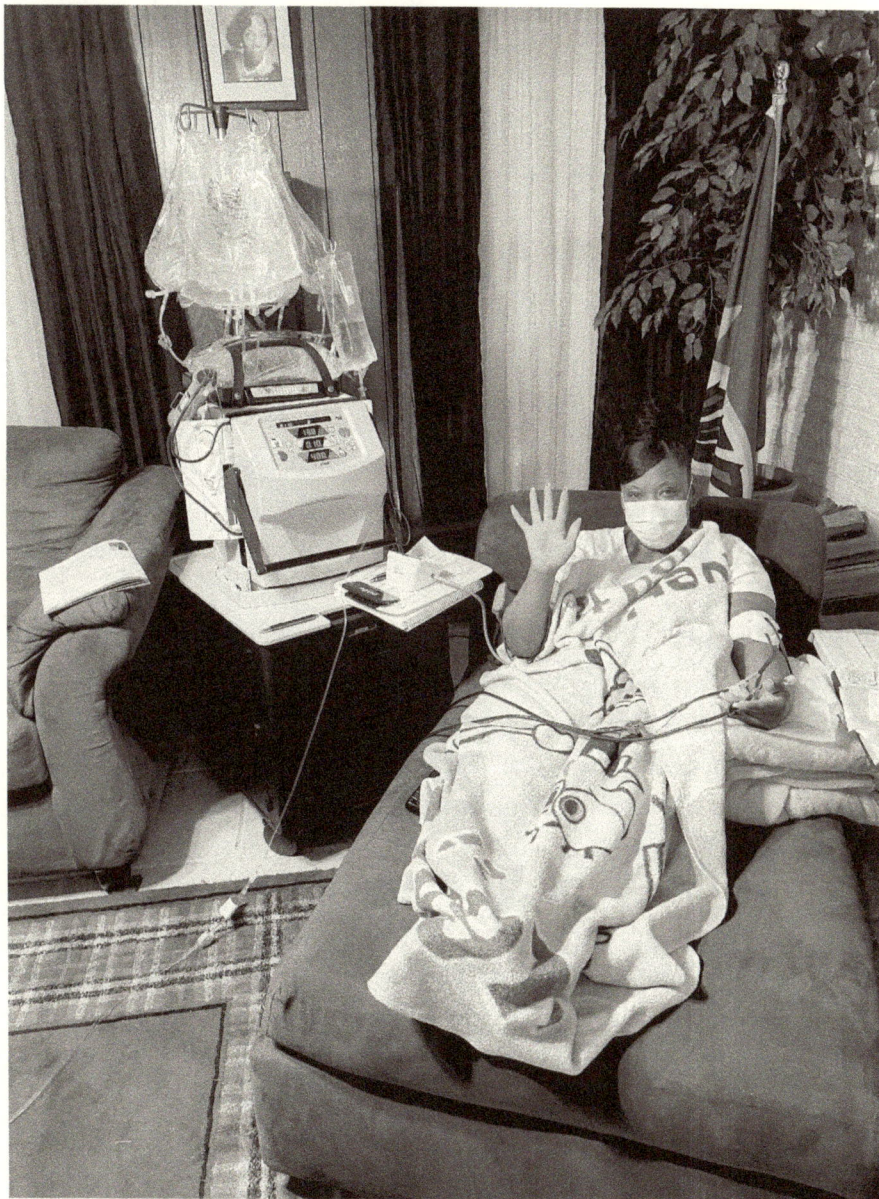

By October 2022, nine months after her diagnosis, the routine of in-center dialysis began to wear on Evette. The early mornings, long sessions, and post-treatment exhaustion weren't just physically draining—they felt like constant reminders of the life she'd lost control over.

She craved more autonomy over her body, her schedule, and her future.

That's when she met Mrs. Harris, the DaVita Spivey Home Dialysis Nurse. Visiting TriCounty regularly to identify potential home dialysis candidates, Mrs. Harris quickly recognized Evette's drive and spirit.

*"You should do this,"* she encouraged. *"It'll give you back so much of your freedom."*

The prospect of managing her treatments at home was both exciting and daunting. But Evette was no stranger to facing challenges head-on. With the support of Mrs. Harris, Leonardo, and her family, she decided to take the leap, determined to reclaim the parts of her life that dialysis had overshadowed.

In November 2022, she and Leonardo began intensive training at DaVita Spivey Home Dialysis Center. Their days still started at 5:00 AM, but this time, every moment was a lesson. From mastering needle placement and machine operation to monitoring vitals and handling emergencies, the learning curve was steep. But Evette and Leonardo approached each challenge as a team, undeterred by the complexities.

Priming the cartridge, preparing the dialysate, assembling the supplies, the *"snap-n-pop"*, addressing alarms and error codes when they occur, and the biggest mental hurdle of them all, self-cannulation—inserting two needles into her fistula for each treatment. The idea of piercing her own skin was overwhelming at first, but with every attempt, her confidence grew.

Leonardo became her steadfast partner, learning the intricacies of the dialysis machine and emergency protocols to ensure Evette's safety. This journey wasn't just hers; it was theirs, and it brought them even closer.

By mid-December 2022, Evette officially transitioned to home dialysis. Each evening, she and Leonardo methodically set up the machine, transforming their home into a space of healing. What once felt like a burden became a routine that granted her the independence she longed for.

Of course, not every session went smoothly. There were times when the machine refused to prime the cartridge correctly—Evette's responsibility—or when the dialysate bag that Leonardo prepared kept throwing error messages. These technical hiccups could test their patience and even spark a little tension between them. But no matter how salty things got, Mrs. Harris was always just a phone call away, ready to troubleshoot and guide them through the mishaps. And though the occasional side-eye or heavy sigh occurred periodically, Leonardo never left Evette's side during a treatment. Even when they were mad at each other, he'd sit there like clockwork—because, after all, who else was going to give her that *"I told you so"* look if something went wrong?

With each passing day, the fear that once accompanied her treatments faded. The needles that once symbolized pain now represented her courage and ability to manage her own care.

No matter how physically demanding the treatments became, Evette refused to let them slow her down. She thrived on movement, on purpose, on keeping her mind engaged even as her body endured the strain of dialysis. Lying still, mindlessly watching television or sleeping through sessions, wasn't an option for her. That kind of passive existence didn't sit right with her spirit. Instead, she treated each treatment as an opportunity—not just to endure but to find new ways to thrive.

She adjusted her routine, weaving productivity into the long hours tethered to the machine. Whether responding to emails, reading articles, or drafting ideas for future projects, she filled the time with intention. If she had to be still, she would still be moving forward. When her body allowed, she stretched, practiced breathing exercises, and even researched ways to strengthen her overall health. She turned her treatments into moments of empowerment rather than limitation.

It wasn't just about keeping busy—it was about reclaiming her time, proving to herself that dialysis wasn't an end but an adjustment. The more she embraced this mindset, the more she realized how much control she still had. She found a rhythm, a balance between self-care and ambition, and that energy radiated outward.

Her determination didn't go unnoticed. Nurses, fellow patients, and even strangers in online support groups took notice of her drive. To them, she became more than just another person undergoing treatment; she became an example of what was possible. She showed them that life didn't have to shrink in the face of illness—it could expand in new and unexpected ways. Dialysis wasn't the end of the road, it wasn't a death sentence. It was just a different route, and Evette was determined to walk it with purpose.

Today, Evette is on the kidney transplant list at Piedmont Hospital, waiting for that transformative call. But regardless of what the future holds, she moves forward with confidence, knowing that she has already reclaimed her life in ways she never thought possible.

# 12

# SCALING NEW HEIGHTS–LIVING FULLY WITH HEMODIALYSIS

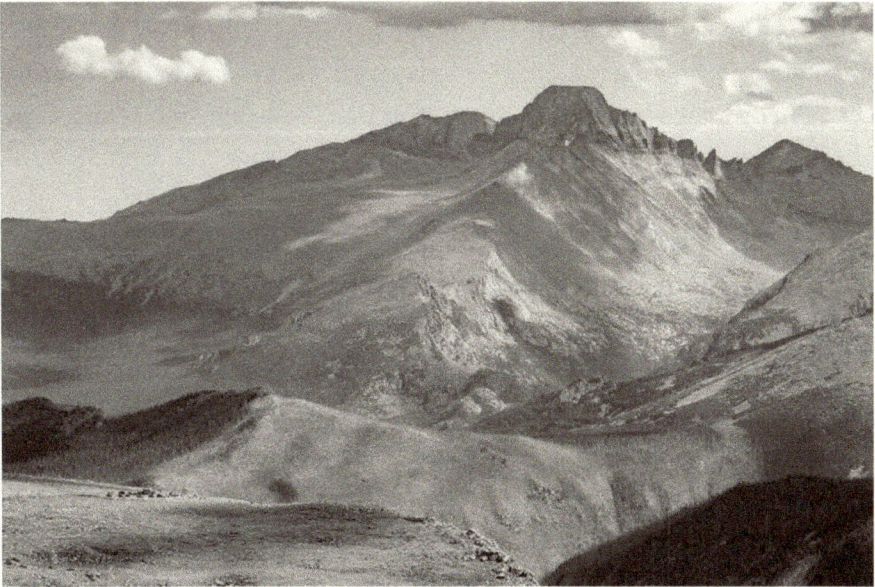

B
y early 2023, with home dialysis now seamlessly integrated into their daily lives, Evette and Leonardo felt prepared to embrace new experiences beyond their usual routine. The opportunity came when Evette was invited to attend a professional conference in Denver, Colorado.

It was the perfect chance to test their new normal in an entirely different environment.

This wasn't their first trip since Evette began dialysis, but it was their first time being away for an entire week and having to travel with "Betsy," the dialysis machine. Packing for the trip was no small feat. NxStage offered two travel case options: a metal case priced around $400 and a soft travel bag for roughly $250. Evette opted for the soft travel case, which looked like an oversized carry-on luggage suitcase with wheels and a handle that slid up in stages for easy transport. She called NxStage directly to place the order and was relieved when the case arrived just in time for their trip.

Mrs. Harris was instrumental in helping them prepare. She coordinated the shipment of medical supplies directly to their hotel in Denver. Once Evette was assigned a hotel room, the staff delivered eight boxes of premixed dialysate— also known as "hanging bags"—and two cartridges to her room, ensuring everything awaited her upon check-in. This thoughtful preparation made the entire process smoother and significantly eased the travel burden.

The medical supplies needed for the week—dialysate, saline, tubing, and sterile dressings—were packed into their own suitcase, which couldn't be carried on. The NxStage machine was checked in as oversized luggage and required special inspection before being loaded onto the plane.

In total, they had six bags: Evette and Leonardo's carry- ons, two suitcases for their personal items, the NxStage machine, and the medical supply bag. Navigating through the airports with so much luggage was tedious, and the oversized baggage check added extra time to their itinerary. But their preparation paid off. The airline was accommodating, and Evette had all the necessary documentation, including a doctor's note explaining the need for the equipment.

Once they arrived in Denver, all the hassle felt worth it. That first evening,

Evette and Leonardo took a leisurely walk through downtown Denver, mar-
veling at the city's impressive skyline. They paused to admire the Colorado
State Capitol Building, noting how much it resembled the Capitol Building
in Atlanta with its striking solid gold dome gleaming under the setting sun.
The comparison sparked a warm conversation about home and the little
similarities that connected distant places.

As they continued their stroll, the crisp mountain air felt different—not
uncomfortable, but noticeably distinct from what they were used to in Georgia.
The altitude gave the evening a unique feel, adding to the novelty of their
adventure.

They eventually found themselves at a nearby Jersey Mike's, craving something simple and familiar. Sitting inside the bustling restaurant, they enjoyed
their sandwiches while people-watching, noting the subtle differences in
how things were done up north. Their conversation flowed easily, filled with
laughter and reflections on their literal and metaphorical journey. It was a
perfect, grounding moment—a reminder that even far from home, they could
find comfort and joy in the simplest of experiences.

Their hotel room became their temporary treatment center. Leonardo easily
set up the machine, transforming a small corner of the room into a healing
space.In addition to attending sessions at the conference, Evette completed
two treatments and still found time to explore the beauty of Denver. The
challenge came the next day when Evette and Leonardo walked 2.5 miles to
the convention center for her first meeting. Although Leonardo accompanied
her, the long walk left Evette feeling exhausted. As Leonardo escorted her
inside, security informed him that he couldn't proceed further without a badge.
Leonardo chuckled and told the officer he wanted to ensure Evette was alright
after the trek.

However, the real challenge awaited inside. The convention center was
massive, and Evette's first meeting was at the far end of the building, up three

long flights of stairs. The higher altitude made her nostrils flare, and it felt as if she'd walked an additional three miles before finally reaching the "*mountain top*," as she humorously dubbed the meeting room for first-time attendees. The room was packed, standing room only, but a kind gentleman noticed her exhaustion and offered his seat. Grateful, Evette relaxed for the hour-long presentation, savoring the chance to catch her breath before heading back to the hotel. She realized then how much the altitude had tested her endurance, but it also gave her a sense of accomplishment—she'd made it through.

Keeping his promise, Leonardo returned an hour later to walk her back to the hotel.

The following morning, realizing the walk was too strenuous to repeat twice daily, Evette quickly pulled out her cell phone and scheduled Ubers for the remainder of the conference. After the first day's challenge, scheduling Ubers transformed the rest of the conference. Whether at the hotel entrance or outside the convention center, her drivers were always prompt, super professional, and consistently earned five- star ratings and generous tips from Evette.

Since their hotel was downtown, they had easy access to various dining options, a nearby mall, and the convenience of room service for breakfast and coffee each morning.

Every day, after her session meetings, they ventured into the city and even took scenic drives through the Rocky Mountains. One day after the conference, they enjoyed a hike up the Cherry Creek Trail and took a tour around the Four Mile Historic Park. The fresh air, the towering peaks, and the stunning landscapes were a refreshing contrast to the clinical environments they were accustomed to. Evette felt alive, and Leonardo was beside her, soaking in every moment.

This trip wasn't just a vacation—it marked a significant milestone in their journey to live fully and embrace new experiences while managing dialysis.

Managing dialysis at home had given Evette back her independence, but traveling with it showed her that the world was still within reach. With careful planning, support from loved ones, and a tenacious spirit, even the most challenging journeys could lead to the most beautiful destinations.

This experience broadened Evette's perspective on what was possible. The confidence she gained from navigating Denver sparked new dreams, and now she and Leonardo are planning their next big adventure—a trip to Europe to celebrate her doctoral graduation!

While traveling with a dialysis machine might seem daunting, Evette and Leonardo's successful journey highlighted how manageable and rewarding it can be. Their story reminds us that life's limitations are often only as big as we allow them to be. With the proper preparation and mindset, living fully while managing hemodialysis isn't just a dream—it's a reality.

# 13

# A TESTAMENT TO ENDURANCE-THE POWER OF PERSEVERANCE

D espite these challenges, Evette has done more than just endure— she has flourished. She has undergone multiple surgeries to comply with her doctors' recommendations, including port catheter surgery, fistula placement surgery, and colorectal surgery. Managing her health requires diligence, as she must keep all medical appointments current and up to date, including vision, dental, mammogram, gynecological, colonoscopy, heart monitoring, and stress tests.

Additionally, she is responsible for drawing and submitting her monthly lab work for both DaVita and Piedmont Hospital. She packages and transports these specimens following the International Air Transport Association (IATA) Dangerous Goods Regulations (DGR) for hazardous materials to ensure compliance. These strict guidelines govern the proper handling, labeling, and transport of biological specimens to maintain safety and integrity throughout the process.

Evette attends monthly medical checkups at DaVita Spivey, where she meets with her dedicated care team. Her nephrologist, Dr. Rahman, is always a familiar face. His children graduated from Woodward Academy and are now pursuing computer science careers. Evette never misses a chance to greet her team with a warm smile and frequently compliments Dr. Rahman on his stylish, designer glasses.

Mrs. Harris, keeps Evette updated on her lab results before each appointment—especially when things aren't looking great. Evette loves to joke with Ms. Harris, teasing her about how quickly she calls when the labs are bad and how quiet things get when the results are good. The home dialysis patients adore Ms. Harris and often feel slighted when she goes on vacation without giving them a heads-up.

To them, she's like family, and many patients, including Evette, prefer not to deal with anyone else. In fact, Evette has personally called Ms. Harris to let her know she'd appreciate being notified in advance if someone else will be filling in when she went on a much-desired vacation in the mountains with her family.

Mrs. Earl, Evette's social worker, is sharp, efficient, and always on top of things. She handles matters quickly and thoroughly and even nominated Evette to serve as the patient representative for their facility's group meetings—a role Evette takes pride in.

The facility's nutritionist, Ms. Mary gives sticker's on the lab report for each component in the normal or above-normal range. She is as kind and sweet as they come, always ready to review lab results with care and adjust medications as needed. Whether it's adding iron, managing medications, or recommending additional testing, Ms. Mary ensures that every patient feels supported and informed.

Ms. Jennifer is the heartbeat of the office, effortlessly keeping everything running like a seasoned office manager. During training, she ensured that Evette and Leonardo had every supply they needed to succeed, setting them up for success each day. Always the first to arrive—often by 4:30 a.m.—she greeted them with her radiant smile and warm spirit, making the early mornings a little easier. Ms. Jennifer plays a vital role at the monthly hemodialysis meetings, ensuring that all patients receive their paperwork, supplies, and medications for their monthly check-ins. She also provides the latest kidney dialysis literature with helpful tips and resources to keep patients informed, empowered, and compliant with their treatment plans.

In the face of these ongoing medical demands, Evette continues to excel in her role at Woodward Academy. She contributes significantly to the institution and is the Junior Varsity Color Guard Faculty Sponsor, inspiring students and colleagues.

Her journey from an unexpected diagnosis to embracing a new normal is a powerful testament to human stamina and the profound impact of unfaltering support from God and loved ones.

# 14

# LOVE & SUPPORT-THE PILLARS THAT HOLD ME UP

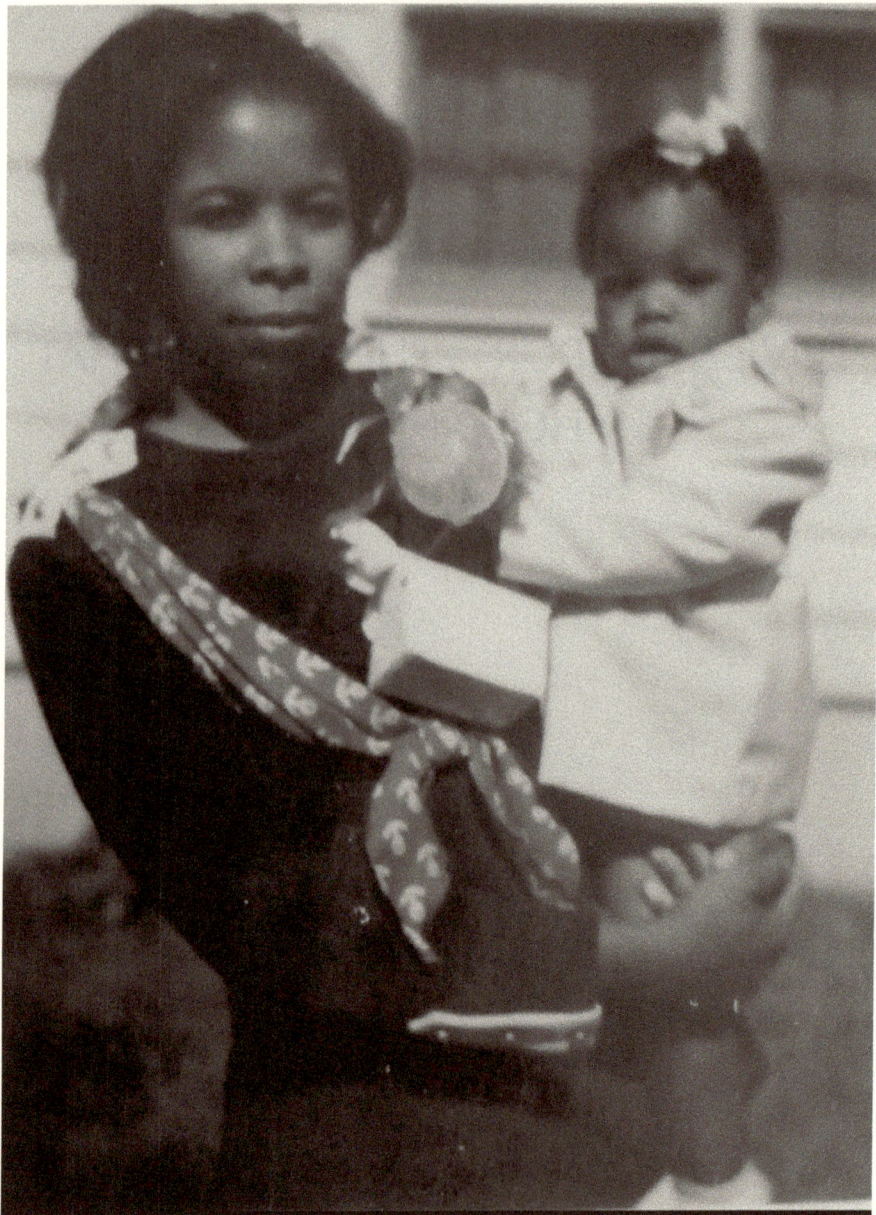

L eonardo is a man shaped by courage and wisdom, hailing from one of Atlanta's known public housing projects. Growing up in the city streets, he forged his strength through life's toughest lessons, becoming a protector by nature. While he wasn't one to show his softer side easily, his love for Evette brought out a tenderness that surprised even him. His family- centered spirit and deep connection with God form the bedrock of their relationship, making him the cornerstone of the life they've built together.

Leonardo often says, "If I'm already there, I don't have to waste time getting there if something goes wrong," a simple statement that embodies his quiet, steadfast presence. Their journey isn't defined by illness but by the relentless bond they've nurtured through every challenge.

But Leonardo wasn't the only source of *unshakable* support in Evette's life. Her mother, Mrs. Fulks, and her father, Officer Scott—affectionately known as "Cigar"—stood as pillars of strength throughout her journey.

Living in South Georgia, Mrs. Fulks a retired Director from the Georgia Department of Revenue, became Evette's spiritual anchor. Though miles apart, her mother's voice brought comfort like no other. Whether through daily phone calls or heartfelt prayers, her powerful spirit remained a beacon of hope. When it came time for Evette's fistula surgery at Emory, Mrs. Fulks made the trip to Atlanta without hesitation, her presence wrapping both Evette and Leonardo in warmth during the stressful days of recovery.

Each day, Mrs. Fulks lifted Evette's name in prayer with her church group, trusting that God would hear their collective voices. Evette often teased her, saying, "*You are one of God's favorites, He spoils you too much!*" With a knowing smile, her mother would reply, "*Evidently, you're one of His favorites too—He's been with you this entire time.*" Those words weren't just comforting; they were a reminder of the divine grace that had carried Evette through each hurdle.

Her father, Officer Scott—"*Cigar*" to those who knew him, a retired Atlanta Police Motorman of 48 years—was the consistent fatherly protector she'd always relied on. Cigar, the quintessential alpha male, had spent years cultivating a tough exterior, rarely letting his emotions show.

But when Evette's health took a turn, that stoicism melted away. His presence was constant, his words of encouragement steady, and his actions spoke volumes about his devotion. *"I don't want to live to see the day something happens to you,"* he told her, his voice soft but firm. *"But I do want to live long enough to see you continue to excel, earn your doctorate, and get that kidney."*

His words weren't just hopes but declarations of his immense pride and love. Witnessing her father transform from a hardened, stoic figure into a source of gentle support was one of the most unexpected and empowering parts of Evette's journey.

Through Leonardo's devotion, her mother's spiritual guidance, and her father's steadfast care, Evette realized she was surrounded by more than just support—she was wrapped in a fortress of love. Their presence wasn't just comforting; it was a testament to the power of family in the face of life's most significant challenges.

Evette's story isn't just one of survival—it's a story of love in its purest form. As she moves forward on her path toward a kidney transplant and her doctorate, she does so with the reassurance of family. The love of those around her isn't just her foundation—it makes her truly *unshakable.*

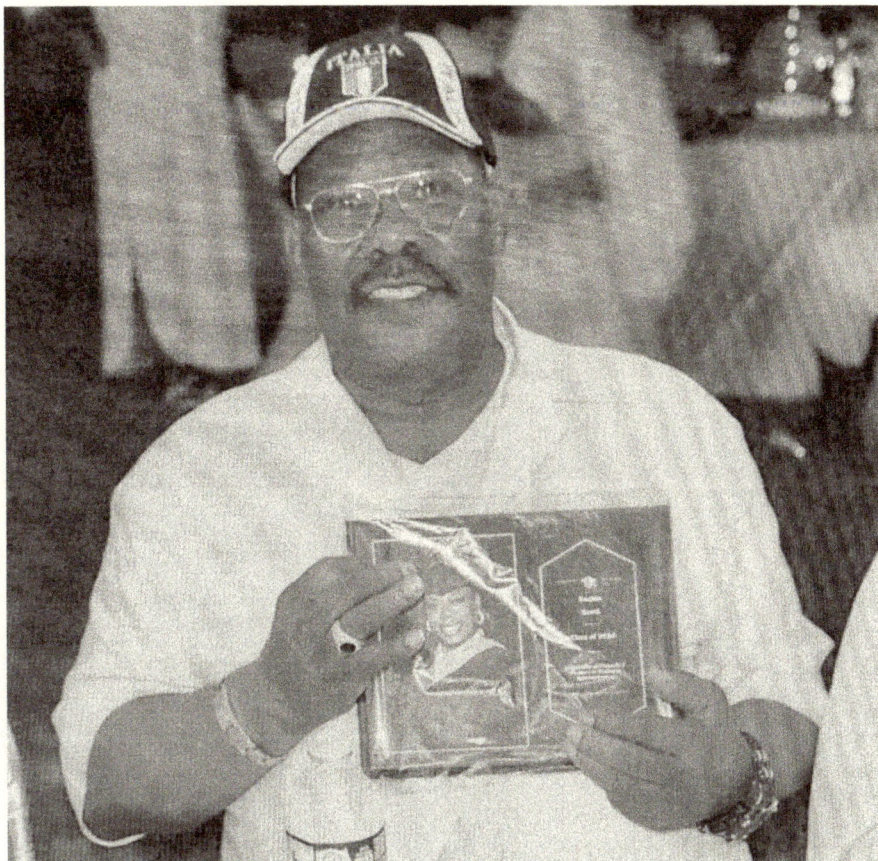

*Officer Scott "Cigar" at the All White Graduation Party!*

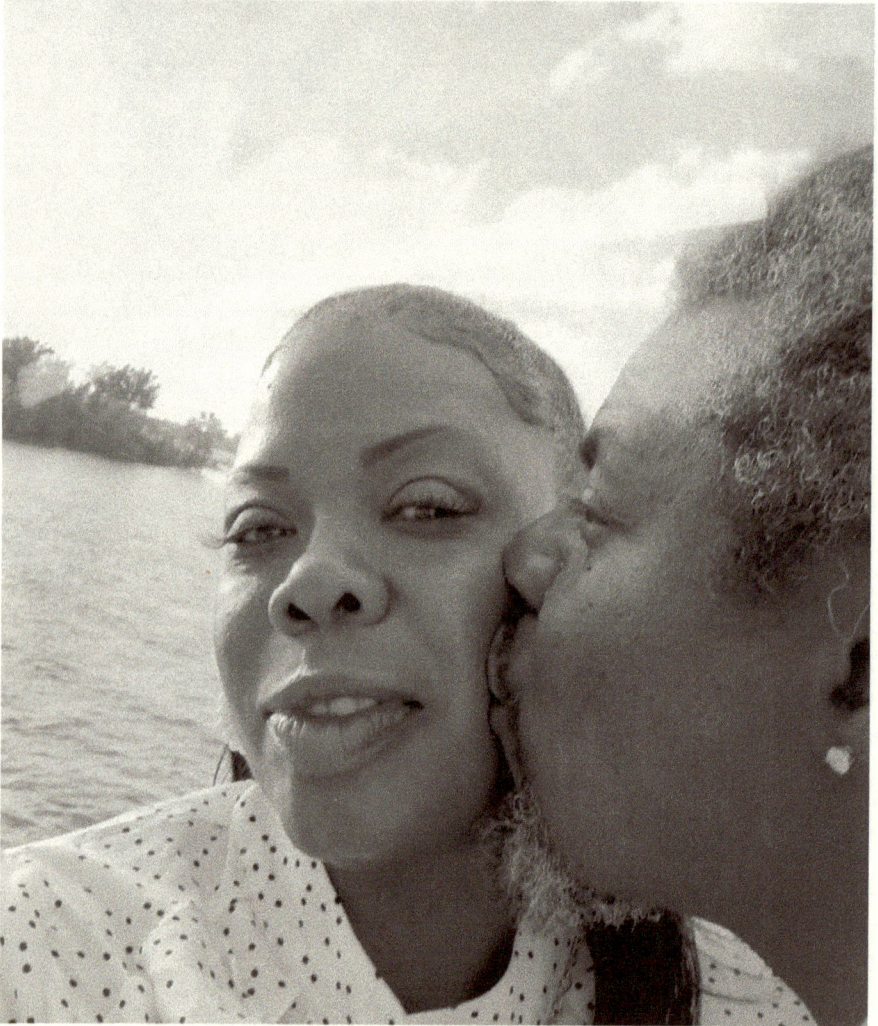

*Evette and Leonardo on the Riverboat at the Canadian Border!*

# 15

# FAITH OVER FEAR-BELIEF IN THE FACE OF THE UNKNOWN

F aith had always been a cornerstone of Evette's life, but her battle with kidney failure strengthened it in ways she never imagined. There were days of frustration—moments when the weight of her condition felt unbearable, when exhaustion clung to her like a second skin—but through it all, she clung to the belief that God had a plan for her. It wasn't blind faith but a deeply rooted conviction shaped by every hardship she'd endured and conquered.

But her trust in that plan was tested in ways she never anticipated. The first time her blood pressure dropped at home during dialysis, Leonardo had to rush to administer saline before she passed out. The first time Evette experienced one of those debilitating cramps during home dialysis, all she could do was lie still until the pain subsided. But the scariest moment for both Evette and Leonardo was when she couldn't stop the bleeding during decannulation at the end of a treatment.

After 45 minutes of applying pressure to her arterial line—the line where unclean blood filters through—the bleeding still wouldn't stop. Normally, it only takes 5 to 10 minutes. Evette softly asked Leonardo to "*call 911.*"

When the ambulance arrived, they sat in the driveway, refusing to enter until the first responders arrived. Leonardo, watching through the front door, saw them idling and his protective instincts kicked in. Evette could hear him cursing from inside the house. When he returned, he explained that EMS couldn't-enter without the first responders, something neither of them had known.

Finally, a fire truck pulled up, and the first responders entered the home. They asked Evette if she could walk while applying pressure to her arm. She nodded, stood up, and was escorted to the gurney outside. Their efforts with gauze and a tourniquet was unsuccessful, the bleeding persisted. It was now 2:00 a.m., and Evette had been bleeding for over an hour. Still, her resolve remained firm. She felt God's presence and wasn't worried—all she wanted was to stop bleeding so she could go to work in the morning.

The EMTs treated her like a gunshot victim and rushed her to Grady Hospital's Trauma Center. In the ambulance, the young EMT was surprised at how calm Evette was, even as her blood pressure remained stable at 115/68. When the EMT checked the bleeding site, a projectile stream of blood shot out. Sirens blared as they sped to the hospital, the EMT tightening the tourniquet even more. Although the pressure from the tourniquet was painful, Evette stayed calm, simply stating, "*I just want to stop bleeding so I can go to work tomorrow.*"

The trauma team sprang into action at Grady—an ER doctor, three nurses, an anesthesiologist, and a surgeon. After 30 minutes of preparation, they cautiously removed the gauze and tourniquet. Amazingly, the bleeding had stopped. Relieved, Evette asked someone to inform Leonardo, who had been anxiously waiting.

The ER doctor explained that repeated cannulation in the same spot had caused scarring and a hole in her fistula, preventing the bleeding from stopping. She would need stitches at the access center and was advised never to use that area again. By 3:15 a.m., Evette was discharged. The next day, unable to go to work, Leonardo took her to the access center, where she received stitches.

These moments were part of the dialysis journey, but what mattered most was the constant assurance that God was always by her side. Evette wasn't worried because she knew deep in her heart that "*God Got This.*" And having Leonardo, her "*Prudential*"—a piece of the rock—by her side made all the difference. Even when life threw the wildest curve balls, she knew he'd be there like clockwork—and probably with a sarcastic comment to lighten the mood.

# 16

# A LEGACY OF STRENGTH–LEAVING A MARK BEYOND ILLNESS

Even now, as Evette continues her journey, she inspires all who meet her. She refuses to allow this illness to define her. Kidney failure may have changed her life, but it never changed her spirit. If anything, it revealed just how strong she truly is.

Each day presents a new set of challenges, yet she meets them with the same quiet determination that has carried her through since the beginning. Some days are harder than others. There are moments of exhaustion, frustration, and questioning—moments where the weight of it all feels overwhelming. But even in those times, she refuses to let doubt take hold. Instead, she leans into her faith, her support system, and her unbreakable resolve to live fully beyond her diagnosis.

Through every challenge, she has demonstrated what it means to persevere. She has proven that hardship doesn't have to weaken you—it can refine you, mold you into someone with greater depth, purpose, and fortitude. The road hasn't been easy, and at times, it has tested her limits. Yet, Evette walks it with grace, never allowing her struggles to diminish her will to push forward.

Home dialysis is more than just a medical treatment—it's a lifestyle shift that demands patience, discipline, and adaptability. The process requires careful attention to detail, strict adherence to medical guidelines, and the presence of a dedicated caregiver to ensure everything runs smoothly.

While dialysis itself isn't fatal, improper treatment—whether from skipping sessions, failing to complete the required treatment time, or mismanaging fluid intake—can have life-threatening consequences. It's not just about staying alive; it's about choosing to fight for more time, more experiences, and more memories.

Leonardo has been Evette's caregiver from the very start. During each home dialysis session, he remains close by, seated on the sofa, watching over her to make sure every setting is correct, every tube is secure, and that she is as comfortable as possible. His quiet presence is a constant reminder of their shared journey—a testament to the power of love and commitment.

Caregiving requires an extraordinary level of patience, sacrifice, and devotion. Leonardo could have chosen distance, allowing fear or fatigue to pull him away. But he didn't. Instead, he stayed, proving that love isn't just about grand gestures or poetic words. It's about showing up—again and again— even when it's hard. It's about holding space for someone's struggle without trying to fix it, about offering strength in the moments when words fail.

Because that's what love looks like.

Because this is what courage looks like.

Because this is what it means to be unshakable.

Evette's journey isn't just about survival—it's about embracing life despite the limitations, about refusing to let her condition dictate her future. She has accepted the uncertainty, the unpredictability, and the raw, unfiltered reality of her health, and in doing so, she has uncovered a resilience that many never realize they possess.

Her story is still being written, but one thing is certain—she will never stop fighting, never stop striving, and never stop inspiring. She has become a beacon of hope for others facing similar battles, proving that even in the face of life's greatest hardships, faith, determination, and the support of loved ones will always triumph.

Her legacy isn't just in the degrees she earns or the milestones she achieves. It's in the lives she touches, the hearts she moves, and the example she sets. She has shown that true strength isn't just about enduring difficulties—it's about doing so with courage, persistence, and an unshakable spirit.

And as she continues forward, one truth remains: Evette's legacy of strength will live on, inspiring generations to come.

# 17

# VICTORY THROUGH ADVERSITY–CELEBRATING RESOLVE IN THE FACE OF KIDNEY FAILURE

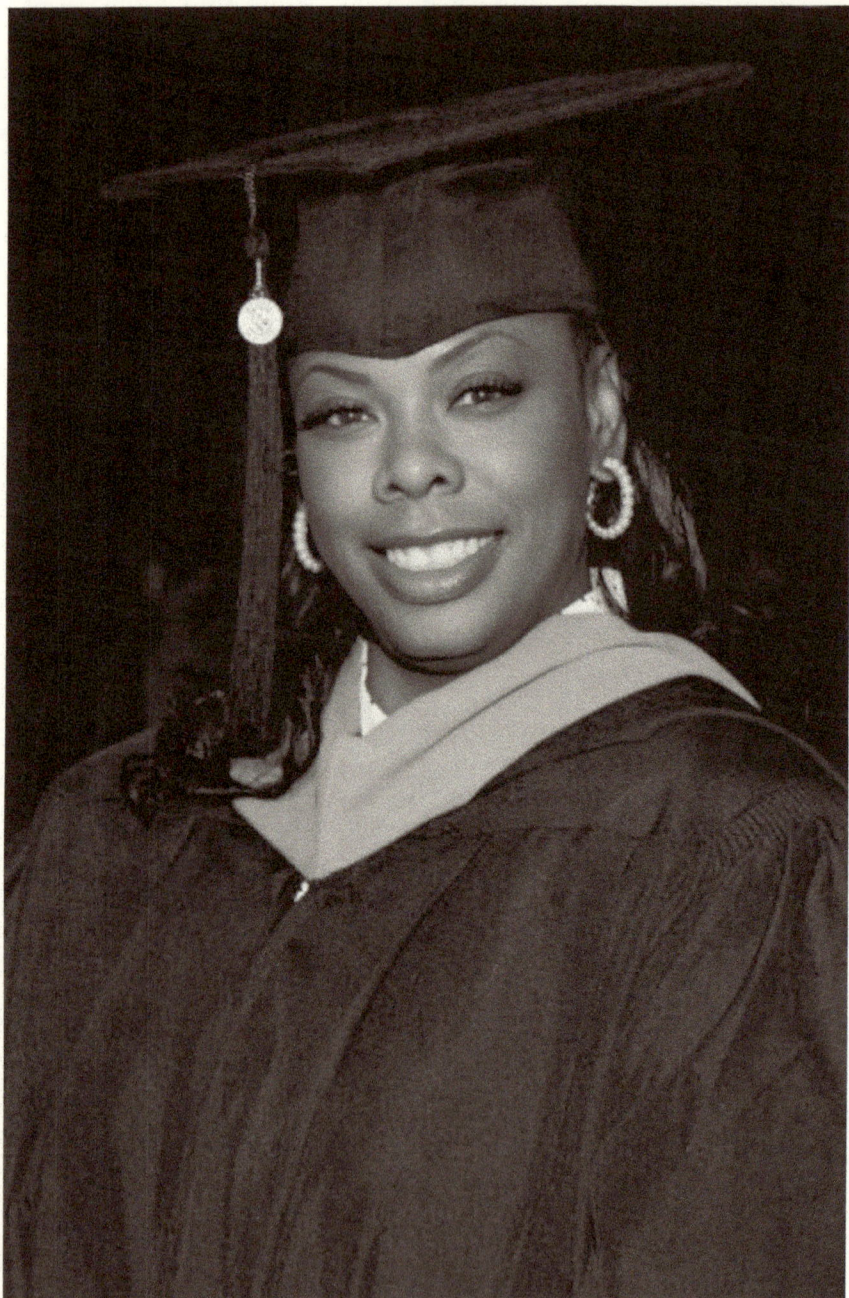

E vette prayed through the difficult moments, giving thanks for the blessings she still had—her family, Leonardo, her career, and the very breath in her lungs. She didn't just pray for healing; she prayed for clarity, patience, and the will to keep moving forward, even when it felt impossible.

Now officially on the kidney transplant list at Piedmont Hospital, Evette waited for the call that could change everything. But she refused to let waiting put her life on hold. Instead of slowing down, she pushed forward, juggling the demands of full-time work, higher education, and her health with an almost relentless determination.

Some mornings, exhaustion weighed so heavily on her that staying in bed seemed like the only reasonable option. But she still got up, dressed, and made her way to campus, forcing herself to push through the fatigue. On days when dialysis left her drained, she masked her discomfort with a practiced smile, greeting colleagues with warmth even when she felt anything but cheerful. She navigated office politics with the same tenacity she applied to her treatments— carefully, strategically, always striving to balance professionalism with the unspoken reality of her condition.

Beyond work, her commitment to her academic goals never faltered. No matter how exhausted she was, she remained focused on earning her Doctorate, determined to cross that finish line despite the toll dialysis took on her body. Even in the midst of it all, she poured energy into her non-profit organization, advocating for K-12 Registrars and fighting for the recognition and resources they deserved.

Evette's life wasn't on pause. If anything, she was moving faster, refusing to let dialysis or the uncertainty of transplant waiting dictate her future. She was still showing up, still chasing dreams, still proving that even in the hardest moments, she was unstoppable, and dedicated to changing her stars.

But for Evette, life wasn't just about pushing through— it was about living fully. If she didn't feel sick, she wasn't going to act sick. She showed up to work with the same energy and professionalism as before, often surprising colleagues who had no idea she was battling a chronic illness. Her ability to maintain a sense of normalcy wasn't just for others—it was a promise she made to herself. She refused to let kidney failure steal her identity.

Balancing dialysis, work, and school wasn't easy. There were days when the fatigue felt like a heavy blanket she couldn't shake off. But Evette found ways to adapt. She became a master of time management, carefully planning her days around treatment schedules and coursework deadlines. She learned to listen to her body, allowing herself rest when needed, but never letting setbacks keep her down for long.

Over time, Evette found herself stepping into a new role: advocate. The support she had received from Lazarus, Mrs. Shirley, Ms. Wanda, and Ms. Winsome inspired her to give back. She became a mentor to new dialysis patients, offering guidance and reassurance to those who felt overwhelmed by their diagnosis. She shared practical tips, like how to manage fluid intake or what to expect during treatments, but she also provided emotional support— reminding others that they were more than their illness.

Her advocacy extended beyond the dialysis center. She began writing about her journey, using her story to raise awareness about chronic kidney disease and the realities of dialysis. It wasn't about seeking sympathy—it was about educating others and breaking down the stigma surrounding chronic illness. Through her words, she offered a window into the everyday challenges and quiet victories of living with kidney disease.

Evette's voice resonated with people far beyond her immediate circle. She was invited to speak at support groups and community events, sharing her journey with honesty and humor. She had a unique ability to make people feel seen and understood, whether they were dialysis patients themselves or loved ones trying to support someone through the process. Her story became a source of encouragement for those facing the overwhelming realities of kidney failure.

But Evette didn't just inspire others—she continued to grow herself. She discovered a deeper sense of purpose in her advocacy, realizing that her journey could be a catalyst for change. She became involved in initiatives aimed at improving patient care and increasing awareness about the importance of organ donation. Her hardiness, combined with her passion for helping others, made her a powerful force in the dialysis community.

Her mantra, *"Faith over fear,"* became more than just words—it was how she navigated every obstacle. Each step forward, no matter how small, was a reminder that while fear might exist, it didn't have the final say. Even on the hardest days, when the exhaustion felt unbearable or the uncertainty of waiting weighed heavily on her heart, Evette chose to believe in the possibility of a brighter future.

Evette's journey wasn't defined by waiting for a transplant—it was shaped by how she chose to live in the meantime. Her strength wasn't just in enduring dialysis; it was in finding purpose and joy despite it. She built a life that was rich with meaning, love, and connection. And in that, she discovered her greatest triumph. Because true victory isn't just about overcoming challenges—it's about progressing in the face of them. And Evette was doing just that, every single day.

# 18

# REFLECTION & WISDOM–LESSONS LEARNED ALONG THE WAY

As Evette settled into life as a dialysis veteran, she became increasingly aware of the shared struggles around her. Kidney failure wasn't just a personal battle—it was a universal one, woven from countless stories of perseverance and hardship. Each face at the dialysis center reflected a journey marked by its own trials, triumphs, and lessons.

Leonardo himself had a family member undergoing in-center dialysis, though his experience starkly contrasted Evette's. This older gentleman had been on dialysis for nearly 20 years, enduring strokes, a heart attack, and grand mal seizures along the way. Yet, he was determined to *live his best life*, unapologetic indulging in cigarettes, weed, beer, and liquor against his doctors' stern warnings. Evette never judged him. Instead, she appreciated their candid conversations, recognizing that everyone coped with illness in their own way.

But there were moments that tested Evette's composure. She knew a young woman with a rebellious streak who defied every medical recommendation— eating what she pleased, skipping treatments, ignoring fluid restrictions and even stopped to dialysis to take a unapologetic approach against her doctor's recommendations which didn't work in her favor. She ended up in the hospital for two weeks, and back on in-center dialysis.

To Evette's disbelief, just two months after their last encounter at a birthday party, the same young woman received *the call* and a kidney transplant. The news stirred a storm of emotions—bitterness, frustration, confusion and jealousy. Here Evette was, meticulously adhering to every guideline, managing her phosphorus levels, limiting her fluids, and attending each dialysis session as prescribed. It felt like an unjust twist in a story she had worked so hard to control.

At her annual kidney transplant follow-up at Piedmont Hospital, Evette finally voiced her frustrations to the transplant social worker—a different face from her trusted Ms. Earl at DaVita Spivey. Letting down her guard, she confessed, *"Maybe I should just allow myself to bleed out and be done with it all."* The words spilled out, raw and unfiltered, spoken from a place of exhaustion and emotional burnout.

But Evette hadn't anticipated the consequences of that moment of vulner-ability. Two months later, she received a call informing her that she had been placed on the *"inactive"* transplant list due to her comments. A mental health evaluation was now required before she could be reactivated. The news blindsided her. She insisted she wasn't suicidal—that her words were a fleeting outburst, not a cry for help. But explanations weren't enough.

Determined to resolve the situation, Evette scheduled a virtual meeting with the transplant psychologist. During the session, she was candid about her anger and jealousy. She didn't sugarcoat her emotions but also made it clear that she had come to terms with them. *"What God has for me is for me,"* she said with conviction. *"That kidney was for her, not me."* It was a turning point. The psychologist saw her not as a risk but as a woman navigating complex emotions with honesty and faith. Shortly after, Evette was reactivated on the transplant list.

In time, Evette found peace with the young woman's journey. She learned that the woman had opened a dance studio, traveled the world, and fully embraced her new life. Rather than harbor resentment, Evette felt genuine happiness for her. It was a moment of profound growth—an understanding that everyone's path unfolds in its own time, guided by forces beyond our control.

This experience deepened Evette's grasp of patience and perspective. She learned that wisdom wasn't just about following the rules; it was about embracing the unpredictability of life, finding grace in the waiting, and trusting in divine timing.

Of course, there were still moments of hesitation. Evette longed to indulge in a glass of wine now and then, but fear held her back. She worried that the moment she allowed herself that simple pleasure, *the call* would come—and she wouldn't be ready. This wasn't just a personal fear; it was rooted in a story Lazarus once shared.

He spoke of a man who, like Evette, had lived a disciplined life on dialysis for 17 years—never drinking, smoking, or straying from medical advice. But on the night of his daughter's high school graduation, he celebrated with one glass of wine. Before he even reached home, *the call* came—a kidney was available. He rushed to the hospital, but when his labs showed traces of alcohol, he was denied the transplant. That single, innocent celebration had cost him the chance at a new life. The story haunted Evette, reinforcing her belief that she needed to be prepared at all times.

With time, Evette began to navigate the dialysis system with the same mindset she applied to every area of her life. She wasn't just attending treatments and monthly follow-ups; she was actively leveraging every available resource to lighten the load and make her journey more manageable. Her experiences transformed her. She was now someone who could offer wisdom, guidance, and hope to others walking similar paths.

Her journey taught her that perseverance wasn't about perfection—it was about persistence. It was about pushing forward even when the road felt unfair, even when others seemed to have it easier. Through it all, her faith remained the anchor that held her steady in life's storms.

Ultimately, Evette learned that life on dialysis wasn't just about surviving—it was about thriving, growing, and embracing the unexpected twists along the way. And as she continued to wait for *the call*, she did so believing her time would come—not a moment too soon, and not a moment too late but right on time.

# 19

# THE POWER OF MOVING FORWARD–EMBRACING LIFE BEYOND DIAGNOSIS

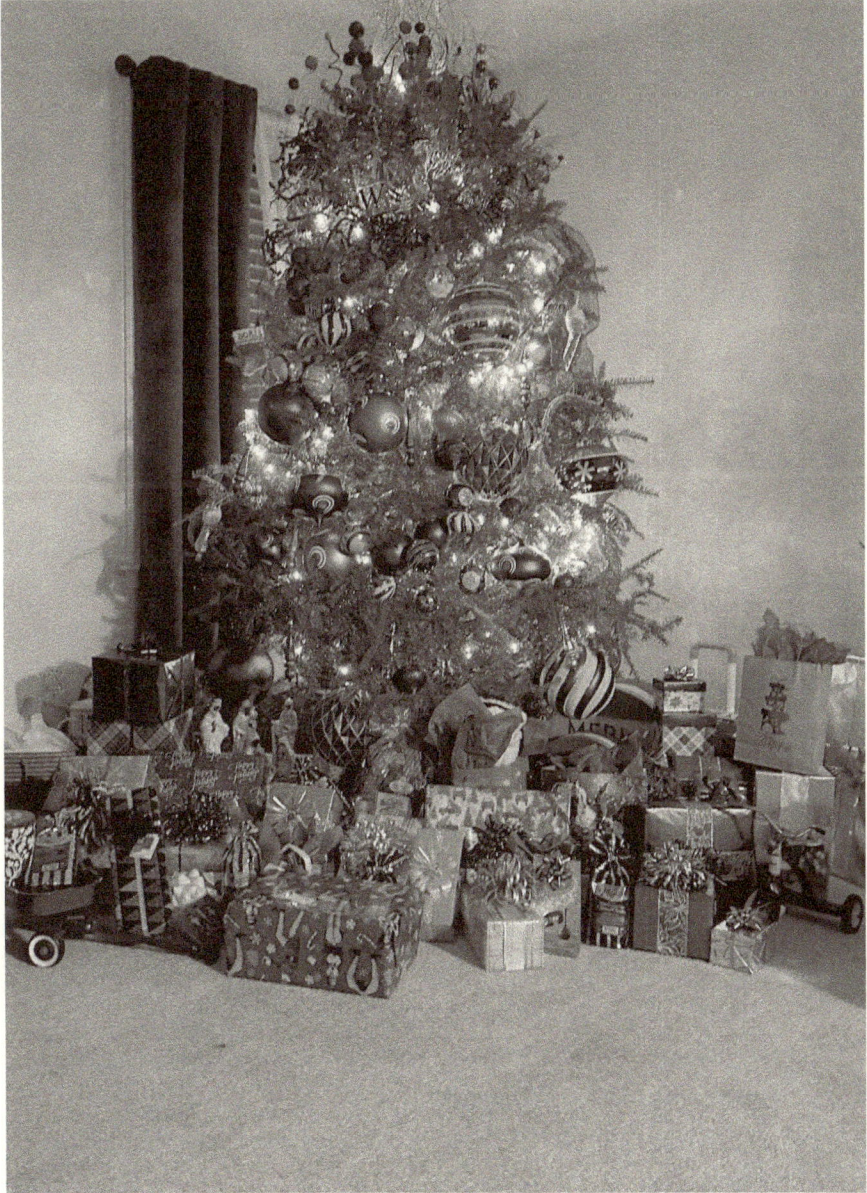

As I close this chapter of my life and this book, I can't help but reflect on how far I've come. When I first started this journey, I never imagined I'd be sharing my story with the world.

In fact, I was hesitant to talk about my condition with anyone beyond my closest circle. Only my parents, children, Leonardo, and my best friend knew what I was going through. I wanted to shield my family from worry, and, truthfully, I wasn't ready to face the reality of my diagnosis out loud.

But something shifted in me. As I grew stronger, I realized that sharing my journey wasn't just about me—it was about offering hope, connection, and inspiration to others. The National Kidney Registry created a website for me to tell my story, and for the first time, I found the courage to put it out on social media. I asked family members to consider being tested for donation, a request that felt vulnerable but necessary.

To my surprise, the support I received was overwhelming. A coworker and three family members reached out on their own, offering to be tested. Their selflessness touched me deeply. I never imagined people would step forward so willingly, and it reinforced the truth that I wasn't in this fight alone.

Prayer groups across the country have kept me in their weekly rotations. My uncle, a pastor of his own church, leads his congregation in lifting my name up to God. Knowing that so many people are praying for me has been a source of immense comfort and strength. Each prayer, each word of encouragement, has been a reminder that my story matters—not just to me, but to everyone who believes in rising above life's toughest hurdles.

Writing this book has been its own journey—a cathartic process that allowed me to confront my fears, celebrate my victories, and reflect on the lessons learned along the way. It hasn't always been easy to put these words to paper, to relive both the darkest moments and the brightest milestones. But in doing so, I've found healing and purpose.

I've learned that healing isn't just physical—it's emotional and spiritual, too. This journey has forced me to face parts of myself I never knew existed. I've discovered courage in the moments I wanted to give up and patience when life didn't move at the pace I hoped for. I've found that sharing my truth, even the messy, uncomfortable parts, connects us in ways that silence never can.

Looking ahead, I know my journey isn't over. There will be new challenges and fresh victories. Life doesn't promise to be easy, but it does promise to be meaningful if we live it with intention, love, and steadfast commitment. I'm ready for whatever comes next because I know I have the tools, the support, and the spirit to face it.

There will be days when doubt creeps in—when the fatigue feels heavier, and the wait for that transplant call feels endless. But I've come to understand that these moments are part of the process. The delays, the frustrations, the unknown—they've all taught me something invaluable: how to find peace even in the waiting. I no longer measure my life by what's missing, but by what's present. And what's present is a whole lot of love, laughter, and purpose.

Though the obstacles are real, I continue to "*live my best life.*" Rollerskating is still one of my greatest joys, feeling the rhythm beneath my feet as I glide across the floor with freedom and grace. Leonardo and I love going fishing, finding peace and connection in nature's quiet embrace. I'm committed to my education, continuing to pursue my Doctorate in Business Administration with the same drive that has carried me through every other part of this journey.

Every year, Leonardo and I host Christmas parties at our home, where the spirit of joy and giving fills every room. We make sure that everyone in attendance leaves with a gift or two. Our gatherings are filled with laughter, games, prizes, and the warmth of shared meals. These moments remind me of the beauty of togetherness and the importance of celebrating life, no matter the circumstances.

Family gatherings are the heartbeat of our lives. We cherish time spent with loved ones, and our home is always filled with the sounds of conversation, music, and love.

Our 2-year-old Belgian Malinois, Shamoo, is the heart of our household. He's so intelligent that he even tries to talk, and his playful spirit brings endless joy to our lives. Watching him grow and learn has been a reminder that life is full of unexpected blessings, even in the smallest moments.

Sometimes, it's the simplest things—like a quiet evening on the porch, a spontaneous road trip with Leonardo, or even just the way Shamoo tilts his head when he doesn't get his way—that remind me how much beauty there is in everyday life. Dialysis may be a part of my routine, but it doesn't own my story. I've learned to find joy not despite my circumstances, but right alongside them.

This story isn't just about kidney failure. It's about the power of pushing past obstacles, the strength of community, and the belief that we can overcome anything. My journey has shown me that we are never alone—and that even in our hardest moments, we have the power to inspire, uplift, and prevail.

So here's to the next chapter—whatever it may hold. I'm ready. And if you're reading this, know that you are, too.

# 20

# A MESSAGE TO YOU, THE
# READER–YOUR JOURNEY STARTS HERE

Share my story and **help me find a kidney**

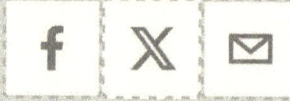

f    X    ✉

See if you're qualified to **donate**

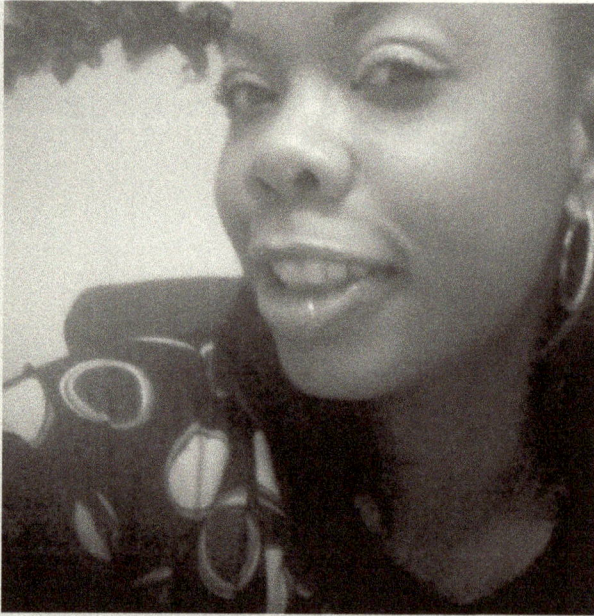

*I am reaching out to seek assistance in finding a kidney donor, a step that would significantly improve my life and allow me to continue pursuing my dreams and passions. My journey with kidney disease has been challenging, but it has also been a testament to resilience and the power of hope.*

🔒 nkr.org

A s you face your own battles—whether it's kidney failure, another illness, or just life throwing its hardest punches—know this: you are more powerful than you realize. The journey may be tough, the nights long, and the path uncertain, but there is strength in every step forward. Even when it feels like you're standing still, you're growing, learning, and becoming more resilient than you were the day before.

It's easy to feel isolated when life doesn't go as planned. I've been there— staring at the ceiling in the middle of the night, wondering *why me?* But what I've learned is that the question isn't *"why me?"*—it's *"what now?"* Life will always present us with challenges we didn't ask for, but it also offers us the courage to rise and the grace to continue.

Don't be afraid to ask for help. Support can come from the most unexpected places. Use your resources. Lean into your circle—whether it's your community, spirituality, family, or even strangers who become friends along the way. I've learned that vulnerability isn't a weakness—it's a bridge to connection and healing. And when you feel like giving up, remember: your story isn't over yet. You are still writing it, day by day. There's more to come, and the best chapters might still be ahead.

*A Reflection on Gratitude*

Through all of this, gratitude has been my anchor. Not the kind of surface-level gratitude where you smile through the pain and pretend everything's okay—but the deep, soul-filling appreciation that comes from knowing you've been through the fire and still managed to rise.

I'm thankful for the prayer groups, both near and far, lifting me in spirit even when I couldn't find the words myself. I'm grateful for the lessons—both the hard ones that knocked me down and the beautiful ones that reminded me to get back up. I've learned to appreciate the silence between storms, the calm after chaos, and the laughter that sneaks in even when life feels overwhelming.

I've discovered that true strength doesn't always roar; sometimes, it's the quiet urge you get to take another step, even when you're exhausted.

Life may have thrown me a curve ball, but it also gave me the tools to hit it out of the park. And for that, I am forever grateful.

## What's Next?

Looking ahead, I'm excited about the future and a life without dialysis. It's not just about waiting for that kidney transplant—it's about living fully in the meantime. We have to remind ourselves constantly that *"this too shall pass."* It's only temporary, and that *"trouble doesn't last always."*

I'm eager to finish my schooling and use my knowledge to create meaningful change in the educational world. I want to advocate for those who don't have a voice, start. But until then, I'm embracing every moment this journey has to offer—living fully, loving fiercely, and continuing to rise. Because life doesn't begin after the transplant; it's happening right now.

## Call to Action: How You Can Make a Difference

If my story has touched your heart, I invite you to take action—not tomorrow, not next week, but today. Consider registering as an organ donor. You could be the reason someone else gets a second chance at life, the answer to prayers whispered in hospital rooms and dialysis centers around the world.

Support organizations like the National Kidney Foundation and the American Kidney Fund, whose work changes lives every single day. These organizations aren't just about statistics and research; they're about people—people like me, people like you, people who are fighting for one more day, one more chance.

Educate your community about chronic kidney disease and the importance of early detection. You never know whose life you might save with a simple conversation.

Every year on my birthday, I use my social media platform to raise money for the National Kidney Foundation. Instead of asking family and friends for personal gifts, I encourage donations directly to the foundation from my page. I don't see the funds, but I see the impact. Each contribution—no matter how small—raises awareness and supports those battling kidney disease.

And if you know someone on dialysis or facing a serious illness, don't just offer to help—show up. A simple message, a listening ear, or a small gesture of kindness can make all the difference. And if you're able, consider being tested as a living donor. You could be the answer to someone's prayers, the light in someone's darkest moment.

Together, we can create a ripple effect of hope, healing, and life. Your actions matter, and you have the power to change lives—starting today.

And so, the journey continues—full of unknowns, possibilities, and everything in between. I'm stepping forward with courage, with promise, and with an open heart. If you're reading this, remember—your story is still being written, and you already hold the strength to embrace whatever comes next.

# 21

# RESOURCES FOR READERS

*Whether you are a patient navigating dialysis, a caregiver supporting a loved one, or simply someone looking to understand more about kidney health, the following resources are designed to offer information, support, and guidance. These organizations, tools, and communities can make a meaningful difference on your journey.*

N**ational Organizations & Foundations National Kidney Foundation (NKF)** *Website:* www.kidney.org

The NKF is one of the leading organizations dedicated to the awareness, prevention, and treatment of kidney disease. They offer educational resources, patient support programs, advocacy opportunities, and up-to-date research on kidney health.

**American Kidney Fund (AKF)**

*Website:* www.kidneyfund.org

AKF provides financial assistance to dialysis patients, offers educational resources on managing kidney disease, and advocates for better care policies. Their website includes tools for understanding treatment options, managing diet, and finding support groups.

**National Kidney Registry (NKR)**

*Website:* www.kidneyregistry.org

The NKR facilitates kidney transplants through donor matching and paired kidney exchanges. Their resources help both patients and living donors navigate the transplant process.

**DaVita Kidney Care**

*Website:* www.davita.com

DaVita offers comprehensive resources for dialysis patients, including treatment options, nutrition guidance,and community support programs.They also provide tools to help you transition from in-center dialysis to home dialysis if it's a suitable option.

### Renal Support Network (RSN)
*Website:* www.rsnhope.org

RSN focuses on inspiring and empowering people living with chronic kidney disease (CKD). They offer peer support, patient advocacy, and educational events to help navigate life with kidney disease.

## *Support Groups & Communities*

### Kidney Disease Support Groups (Online & Local)
*Find local groups through:*

- Your dialysis center or hospital
- National Kidney Foundation support group directory
- Facebook groups and online forums dedicated to kidney disease and dialysis

## *Transplant Communities*

Connecting with others who have undergone kidney transplants can offer valuable insights and emotional support. Many transplant centers have their own peer support programs or can connect you with mentors who've been through the process.

## *Caregiver Support*

### Family Caregiver Alliance:
www.caregiver.org

Offers resources for those caring for individuals with chronic illnesses, including emotional support and practical care giving tips.

# 22

# PRACTICAL TIPS FOR DIALYSIS WARRIORS

*Navigating dialysis and chronic kidney disease (CKD) can be overwhelming, but with the right tools and resources, you can take charge of your health and well-being. Whether you're newly diagnosed or a kidney disease patient, these practical tips, apps, and resources will help you stay informed, organized, and empowered.*

## Staying Organized & Managing Treatments

· **My DaVita App**

Track your treatments, medications, lab results, and appointments. This app helps dialysis patients monitor fluid intake, manage dietary restrictions, and connect with their care teams for personalized support.

· **Digital Planners& Health Trackers**

Use tools like Google Calendar or health tracking apps to log your dialysis schedule, medications, and doctor visits.

Keeping a routine helps manage treatments more efficiently.

· **Prepare for Emergencies**

Always have an emergency kit at home that includes essential medical supplies, a list of medications, and instructions for loved ones in case of complications during treatment.

## Managing Your Diet & Nutrition

· **Kidney Disease Diet Apps**

Apps like Google Calendar and My Kidney Coach provide personalized dietary guidance, recipe ideas, and nutritional tracking to help maintain a kidney-friendly diet.

- **Communicate with Your Nutritionist**

Build a strong relationship with your nutritionist to understand your specific dietary needs, including managing sodium, potassium, phosphorus, and fluid intake.

## Financial & Legal Resources

- **Patient Assistance Programs**

**American Kidney Fund Financial Assistance**: Offers help with treatment-related costs.

**NeedyMeds**: www.needymeds.org for information on assistance programs for medications and healthcare expenses.

## Understanding Insurance & Medicare

- **Medicare Coverage for Dialysis &Transplant Services**: Visit www.medicare.gov for detailed explanations of services covered under Medicare for kidney patients.
- **State Assistance Programs**: Check with your state's health department for additional coverage options and financial support.

## Employment Rights for Dialysis Patients

- **Family Medical Leave Act (FMLA)**: Know your rights when balancing work and dialysis. FMLA offers protections for medical leave, including intermittent leave when needed.
- Americans with Disabilities Act (ADA): Understand your legal protections

regarding reasonable accommodations in the workplace.

## Emotional Well-Being & Support Systems

### · Prioritize Mental Health

It's normal to feel overwhelmed. Consider talking to a counselor, therapist, or trusted friend to process your emotions. Many dialysis centers offer access to social workers who can provide emotional support.

### · Find Support

Connect with other dialysis patients through support groups or online communities. Sharing experiences offers comfort, advice, and the reassurance that you're not alone.

## Educational Resources& Reading

### · Books on Kidney Health& Resilience:

*Coping with Kidney Disease: A 12-Step Treatment Program to Help You Avoid Dialysis* by Mackenzie Walser

*The Patient's Guide to* Dialysis by Rich Snyder, DO

*The Courage to Keep Going: Inspiring Stories from Kidney Disease Survivors* (Various Authors)

· Webinars & Podcasts:

*The Kidney Cast*: A podcast sharing personal stories from people living with kidney disease and transplants.

**NKF Webinars**: Educational sessions from the National Kidney Foundation, covering everything from managing CKD to preparing for a transplant.

## For Potential Donors & Advocates

- **Becoming a Living Donor:**

**National Kidney Registry's Donor Information**: Learn about the living donor process,eligibility, and how you can potentially save a life.

**OrganDonor.gov**: The official U.S. government site for registering as an organ donor.

## Advocacy & Volunteering:

Join advocacy efforts to improve kidney care policies, increase awareness, and support research. Many of the organizations listed above have advocacy programs you can participate in.

## *Final Words of Encouragement Celebrate Small Wins*

*Every milestone—big or small—is a victory.*

*Acknowledge your progress and give yourself grace on tough days.*

*Remember, You're Not Alone*

Lean into your support systems, stay informed, and hold onto hope. Whether you are newly diagnosed, a long-time dialysis patient, or a caregiver, staying connected and informed empowers you to make the best decisions for your health.

If you're looking for more personalized support, reach out to your healthcare team, social workers at your dialysis center, or trusted friends and family. There is strength in connection, and together, we can navigate the challenges and celebrate the victories.

# 23

# GLOSSARY OF MEDICAL TERMS

**A**rterial Line: A tube inserted into an artery, often used during dialysis to carry blood from the patient to the dialysis machine for filtering.

**Chronic Kidney Disease (CKD)**: A progressive condition where the kidneys gradually lose their ability to filter waste and excess fluids from the blood over time.

**Creatinine**: A waste product from normal muscle breakdown that is filtered out by healthy kidneys. Elevated levels in the blood indicate impaired kidney function.

**Dialysate**: A special fluid used in dialysis to help remove waste, toxins, and extra fluid from the blood.

**Dialysis**: A life-sustaining treatment that takes over the kidneys' job of removing waste, toxins, and excess fluid from the bloodstream when kidney function is severely reduced.

**End-Stage Renal Disease (ESRD)**: The final, most severe stage of chronic kidney disease, where kidney function has declined so much that dialysis or a kidney transplant is required to sustain life.

**Fistula**: A surgically created connection between an artery and a vein, usually in the arm, that provides easy access for inserting dialysis needles.

**Focal Segmental Glomerulosclerosis (FSGS)**: A type of kidney disease characterized by scarring in parts of the kidneys' filtering units (glomeruli), leading to protein leakage in the urine and potential kidney failure.

**Hemodialysis**: A type of dialysis where a machine filters waste, toxins, and excess fluids directly from the blood through a vascular access point like a fistula or catheter.

**Home Hemodialysis**: A form of hemodialysis performed at home, allowing patients greater flexibility and control over their treatment schedule.

**Intermittent Family Medical Leave (FMLA)**: A legal protection allowing employees to take unpaid, job-protected leave for medical conditions, including dialysis treatments, on an as-needed basis.

**Nephrologist**: A doctor who specializes in diagnosing and treating kidney diseases and managing dialysis and transplant care.

**Peritoneal Dialysis**: A type of dialysis where a cleansing fluid is introduced into the abdominal cavity, allowing waste products to be drawn out through the lining of the abdomen(peritoneum) before being drained.

**Port Catheter (Central Venous Catheter)**: A temporary device inserted into a large vein in the neck, chest, or groin, providing immediate access for hemodialysis.

**Proteinuria**: The presence of excessive protein in the urine, often a sign of kidney damage.

**Saline Flush**: A sterile saltwater solution used in dialysis to maintain blood pressure stability and clear lines when blood pressure drops during treatment.

**Self–Cannulation**: The process where dialysis patients insert their own needles into their fistula or graft for treatment, offering greater independence and control.

**Transplant List**: The official registry of individuals awaiting organ transplants, prioritized based on medical urgency and compatibility.

**Uremia**: A serious condition where waste products build up in the blood due to kidney failure, leading to symptoms like fatigue, nausea, confusion, and shortness of breath.

**Venous Line:** The venous line is part of the extra corporeal circuit, carrying filtered blood from the dialysis machine back into the patient's bloodstream. It works in conjunction with the arterial line, which draws blood from the body for filtration.

# 24

# References

American Kidney Fund. (n.d.). *Living with kidney disease.* https://w
ww.kidneyfund.org/kidney-disease/kidney-failure/living-kidney-
failure

Centers for Disease Control and Prevention. (2022).*Chronic kidney disease basics.* https://www.cdc.gov/kidneydisease/basics.html

DaVita Kidney Care. (n.d.).*Understanding dialysis treatment options.* Retrieved from https://www.davita.com/treatment-options

Family Caregiver Alliance. (n.d.). *Caring for a loved one with chronic illness.* https://www.caregiver.org

Mayo Clinic.(2023). *Focal Segmental Glomerulosclerosis (FSGS).* https://www.m ayoclinic.org/diseases-conditions/fsgs

Minter, K. (2024). *Harnessing equity in education: Empowering students of color in education.* NAIS National People of Color Conference, Denver, CO. Woodward Academy.

National Kidney Foundation. (n.d.).*Chronic kidney disease (CKD).* https://www.

kidney.org/atoz/content/about-chronic-kidney-disease

National Kidney Registry. (n.d.). *Understanding dialysis and transplantation.* https://www.kidneyregistry.org/understanding-dialysis-and-transplantation

NeedyMeds. (n.d.).*Assistance programs for medications and healthcare costs.* https://www.needymeds.org

Renal Support Network. (n.d.). *Patient support and advocacy resources.* https://www.rsnhope.org

U.S. Department of Health and Human Services. (n.d.). *Organ donation and transplantation resources.* https://www.organdonor.gov

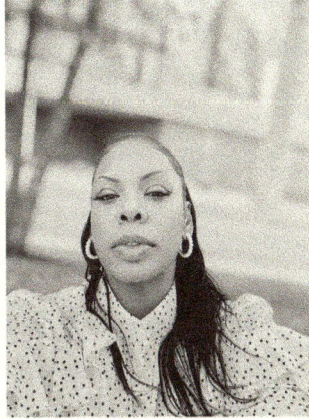

# About the Author

Kechia Scott is a passionate advocate, educator, and author whose journey with chronic kidney disease (CKD) and dialysis has inspired countless individuals to find strength in adversity. A native of Atlanta, Georgia, her story is one of resilience, faith, and an unwavering commitment to living life on her own terms.

As the Registrar at Woodward Academy in College Park, Georgia—the largest private school in the continental United States—Kechia plays a pivotal role in maintaining academic records and supporting students and faculty. Her professional background reflects a commitment to excellence, organization, and fostering a supportive academic environment. Despite balancing a demanding career with her health challenges, she remains a model of perseverance in the face of life's toughest trials.

Kechia holds a Bachelor's degree in Business Management, a Master of Business Administration (MBA), and is currently pursuing her Doctor of Business Administration (DBA) at the University of Phoenix. Her doctoral research focuses on the lack of certification standards for K-12 Registrars, highlighting her dedication to education, professional development, and advocacy for the field.

Her personal journey with kidney failure, dialysis, and the path to a transplant has been both challenging and transformative. Through it all, she has become a beacon of hope in the dialysis community—mentoring fellow patients, sharing her experiences in support groups, and advocating for kidney disease awareness. Her work has been featured through the National Kidney Registry, and in 2024, she was selected to present at the National Association of Independent Schools (NAIS) People of Color Conference, where she led a workshop on leveraging data to empower students of color.

Kechia's life is enriched by the unwavering love and support of her family, including her steadfast partner, Leonardo, her children, and her parents, who have been pillars of strength throughout her health journey. She finds joy in roller skating, fishing, and hosting her annual Christmas parties, filled with laughter, games, and generosity. Adding to her daily moments of joy is Shamoo, Leonardo's loyal Belgian Malinois, whose presence brings lightheartedness and companionship.

Through her book, Unshakable, Kechia offers more than just her personal story—she delivers a powerful message of hope, perseverance, and community. She aims to educate, uplift, and inspire those navigating similar challenges, proving that a diagnosis is not a death sentence. Instead, it is an opportunity to recharge, restructure, and embrace new beginnings.

Looking ahead, Kechia plans to expand her advocacy by speaking publicly about kidney health, dialysis, and the importance of early detection. She dreams of growing her non-profit organization for K-12 Registrars, traveling, completing her doctorate, and broadening her impact in both education and healthcare. Her ultimate goal is simple but profound: to inspire others to face life's challenges head-on, with courage, resilience, and an unshakable spirit.

**You can connect with me on:**

🔲 https://facebook.com/kechiam

🔗 https://www.linkedin.com/in/kechia-minter-749027173

**Subscribe to my newsletter:**

✉ https://substack.com/@kvette71

www.ingramcontent.com/pod-product-compliance
Lightning Source LLC
Chambersburg PA
CBHW021148090426
42740CB00008B/1006